MW01714096

REFLEXOLOGY

AND

AROMATHERAPY

BIBLE

BY

Toni Austin

Terms and Conditions

LEGAL NOTICE
(BLP01072016)

The Publisher has strived to be as accurate and complete as possible in the creation of this report, notwithstanding the fact that he does not warrant or represent at any time that the contents within are accurate due to the rapidly changing nature of the Internet.

While all attempts have been made to verify information provided in this publication, the Publisher assumes no responsibility for errors, omissions, or contrary interpretation of the subject Matter herein. Any perceived slights of specific persons, peoples, or organizations are unintentional.

In practical advice books, like anything else in life, there are no guarantees of income made. Readers are cautioned to reply on their own judgment about their individual circumstances to act accordingly.

FREE GIFT FROM THE PUBLISHER

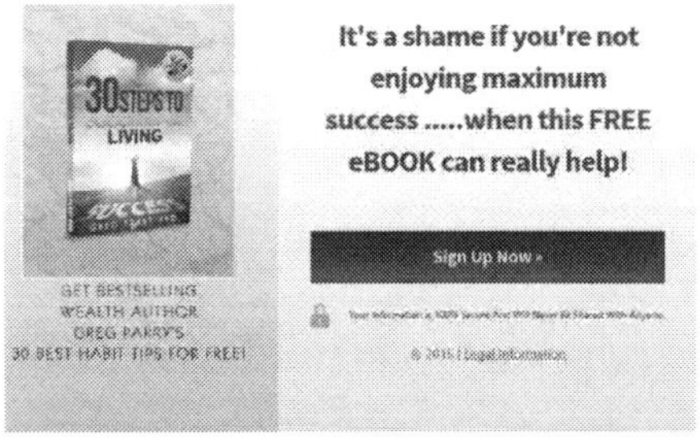

Please search this page www.onelifeblog.com/free-success-guide

BOOK 1
REFLEXOLOGY

BOOK 2
AROMATHERAPY

REFLEXOLOGY AND AROMATHERAPY BIBLE By Toni Austin

Table of Contents

BOOK 1 REFLEXOLOGY

History of Reflexology

Modern reflexology is based on an ancient form of therapy. There is evidence of some form of foot and hand therapy being Practised in China as long ago as 4,000 B.C. and also at the same time in Egypt, as depicted in the tomb of Ankmahor. The North American tribes of Indians are known to have Practised a form of foot therapy for hundreds of years.

There is some confusion about the true origin of this powerful therapy, sufficient to say that it has stood the test of time and has helped thousands of people to better health.

The dictionary definition of a "Reflex" is "an involuntary or instinctive movement in response to a stimulus" or in the sense of reflection or mirror image.

The reflexes on our feet and hands act as mirror images of the body.

Zone Therapy was used as far back as AD1500. The American president, James Abram Garfield was said to apply pressure to his feet to relieve pain.

During the 16th Century a number of books were published on Zone Therapy, one was written by Dr Adamus and Dr A'tatis and another by Dr Ball in Leipzig.

The re-discovery of some form of systemized foot treatment is accredited to Dr. William Fitzgerald who called it Zone Therapy and drew it to the attention of the medical world between 1915 and 1917. It was in 1915 that an article entitled "To stop that toothache, squeeze your toe" was published in "Everybody's Magazine", written by Edwin Bowers, which first brought Dr. Fitzgerald's work on Zone Therapy before the public.

In 1917, Dr. Fitzgerald wrote "Zone Therapy or Relieving Pain in the Home". Two years later, they enlarged this book and published it under a second title "Zone Therapy or Curing Pain and Disease".

Dr. William Fitzgerald (1872 – 1942) received his medical degree from the University of Vermont in 1895. He practiced in Boston City Hospital for two and a half years before going to London. He spent two years at the Central London Nose and Throat hospital before taking up a position in Vienna as Assistant to Professors Politzer and Chiari, who were highly respected doctors.

Dr. Ada Politzer (1835 – 1920) of the University of Vienna, was a well-known author of many medical books and made clinical contributions to the diagnosis and treatment of diseases of the ear. Dr. Otto Chiari, again an established authority, wrote several books on diseases and surgery of the larynx and trachea.

Dr Fitzgerald never published the original sources for his own therapy, but it is likely that he was influenced during this time in Vienna, by the work of Dr. d'Arsonval. In "Zone Therapy is Scientific" by Dr W D Chesney, it is stated that in Germany, Dr. d'Arsonval was using physiotherapy and getting relief following the use of reflex knowledge which, in effect, was what was later termed Zone Therapy by Drs Fitzgerald and Bowers.

When Dr Fitzgerald returned to the United States, he became head of the Nose and Throat Department at St Francis Hospital, Hartford, Connecticut. Around 1909, Dr Fitzgerald discovered, or re-discovered Zone Therapy. Almost ten years later, he wrote his book, about how he had stumbled upon the concept of Zone Therapy:

"Six years ago I accidentally discovered that pressure with a cotton tipped probe on the muco-cutinous margin (where the skin joins the mucous membrane) of the nose gave an anaesthetic result as though a cocaine solution had been applied. I further found that there were many spots in the nose, mouth, throat and on both surfaces of the tongue, which, when pressed firmly, deadened definite areas of sensation. Also, that pressure exerted over any bony eminence of the hands, feet or over the joints, produces the same characteristic results in pain relief. I found also that when pain was relieved, the condition that produced the pain was most generally relieved. This led to my 'mapping out' these various areas and their associated connections and also to noting the conditions influenced through them. This science I have named "Zone Therapy".

It is worth noting that the Chinese had, in acupuncture, divided the body into longitudinal meridians by approximately 2,500 B.C.

From 1915 and into the early 1930's, the subject of zone therapy was controversial, although it met with a certain amount of success with osteopaths and dentists.

One physician who did believe in Fitzgerald's work was Dr. Joe Shelby Riley of Washington. He and his wife, Elizabeth, credit Dr. Fitzgerald as one who, in modern times, brought this science (ie. Zone therapy) to the notice of the public.

The physiotherapist working with Dr. Riley at St Petersburg, was Eunice Ingham (1889 – 1974). Eunice Ingham extended the work of Dr. Fitzgerald and painstakingly mapped the feet with all the corresponding organs and glands of the body. She was a real pioneer who was determined to help people to help themselves, if their doctor was not using reflexology. In the early years, she worked with doctors to prove her findings and to demonstrate to them that reflexology was a useful diagnostic tool.

She lectured at a medical clinic headed by Dr. Charles Epstein in May 1939. In his report, he acknowledged that reflexology worked. However, while they knew it worked, doctors were not interested in using it, because reflexology was too time consuming and they could not make as much money.

Eunice Ingham is still known as the pioneer of modern reflexology and she authored two well-known books "Stories the Feet Can Tell" and "Stories the Feet Have Told". They have since been combined into one volume. In addition to her writing and lecturing, she, along with her nephew, Dwight Byers, founded the International Institute so that her work could be continued in perpetuity.

Dwight Byers is the current President of the Institute. He worked for many years with his Aunt and is equally keen that her work and that developed by the Institute more recently, should be passed on for the benefit of many people.

Throughout her forty years of experience treating many thousands of people, Eunice Ingham devised a system of techniques which enable the practitioner to contact the reflexes in the most effective and economic way. This system is known as the "Original Ingham Method" and though this method has been refined still further through research by Dwight Byers and staff at the Institute, her legacy is still thoroughly entwined in the practical techniques that we teach.

The years of World War II interrupted Eunice Ingham's travelling for a time, but in 1947 she was joined on her lecture tour by her nephew. Each of Eunice Ingham's seminars was unique. Her method of instruction was to demonstrate and lecture as she worked on the health problems of those who attended. Over the years, Dwight Byers has contributed to his aunt's work by organizing the seminars into training workshops. These have been further developed to produce the Diploma course that we teach in the UK.

Eunice Ingham died in 1974, having devoted forty years of her life to reflexology. Today, her legacy continues and she would be proud to see how reflexology has been developed into a profession. So those of us associated with the International Institute of Reflexology are indeed fortunate that we have the opportunity to get so close to the originator of the techniques.

Reflexology can benefit people of all ages and, depending on the length of time a condition has been present, can improve or eliminate many ailments during a course of four to six weekly treatments.

REFLEXOLOGY AND AROMATHERAPY BIBLE By Toni Austin

Foreword

Reflexology may be defined as a practice of applying pressure to the feet and hands using thumb, finger, and hand techniques without the use of oils, creams, or lotions. Based on a system of zones, that reflects an image of the body on the feet and hands which in turn effects the physical changes made in the body.

Definition

Reflexology is a therapeutic method of relieving pain by stimulating predefined pressure points on the feet and hands. This controlled pressure alleviates the source of the discomfort. In the absence of any particular malady or abnormality, reflexology may be as effective for promoting good health and for preventing illness as it may be for relieving symptoms of stress, injury, and illness.

Reflexologists work from maps of predefined pressure points that are located on the hands and feet. These pressure points are reputed to connect directly through the nervous system and affect the bodily organs and glands. The reflexologist manipulates the pressure points according to specific techniques of reflexology therapy. By means of this touching therapy, any part of the body that is the source of pain, illness, or potential debility can be strengthened through the application of pressure at the respective foot or hand location.

Purpose

Reflexology promotes healing by stimulating the nerves in the body and encouraging the flow of blood. In the process, reflexology not only quells the sensation of pain, but relieves the source of the pain as well.

Anecdotally, reflexologists claim success in the treatment of a variety of conditions and injuries. One condition is fibromyalgia. People with this disease are encouraged to undergo reflexology therapy to alleviate any of a number of chronic bowel syndromes associated with the condition. Frequent brief sessions of reflexology therapy are also recommended as an alternative to drug therapy for controlling the muscle pain associated with fibromyalgia and for relieving difficult breathing caused by tightness in the muscles of the patient's neck and throat.

Reflexology applied properly can alleviate allergy symptoms, as well as stress, back pain, and chronic fatigue. The techniques of reflexology can be performed conveniently on the hand in situations where a session on the feet is not practical, although the effectiveness of limited hand therapy is less pronounced than with the foot pressure therapy.

Description

Origins

Reflexology is a healing art of ancient origin. Although its origins are not well documented, there are reliefs on the walls of a Sixth Dynasty Egyptian tomb (c. 2450 B.C.) that depict two seated men receiving massage on their hands and feet. From Egypt, the practice may have entered the Western world during the conquests of the Roman Empire. The concepts of reflexology have also been traced to pre-dynastic China (possibly as early as 3000 B.C.) and to ancient Indian medicine. The Inca civilization may have subscribed to the theories of reflexology and passed on the practice of this treatment to the Native Americans in the territories that eventually entered the United States.

In recent times, Sir Henry Head first investigated the concepts underlying reflexology in England in the 1890s. Therapists in Germany and Russia were researching similar notions at approximately the same time, although with a different focus. Less than two decades later, a physician named William H. Fitzgerald presented a similar concept that he called zone analgesia or zone therapy. Fitzgerald's zone analgesia was a method of relieving pain through the application of pressure to specific locations throughout the entire body. Fitzgerald divided the body into 10 vertical zones, five on each side, that extended from the head to the fingertips and toes, and from front to back. Every aspect of the human body appears in one of these 10 zones, and each zone has a reflex area on the hands and feet. Fitzgerald and his colleague, Dr. Edwin Bowers, demonstrated that by applying pressure on one area of the body, they could anesthetize or reduce pain in a corresponding part. In 1917, Fitzgerald and Bowers published Relieving Pain at Home, an explanation of zone therapy.

Later, in the 1930s, a physical therapist, Eunice D. Ingham, explored the direction of the therapy and made the startling discovery that pressure points on the human foot were situated in a mirror image of the corresponding organs of the body with which the respective pressure points were associated. Ingham documented her findings, which formed the basis of reflexology, in Stories the Feet Can Tell, published in 1938. Although Ingham's work in reflexology was inaccurately described as zone therapy by some, there are differences between the two therapies of pressure analgesia. Among the more marked differences, reflexology defines a precise correlation between pressure points and afflicted areas of the body. Furthermore, Ingham divided each foot and hand into 12 respective pressure zones, in contrast to the 10 vertical divisions that encompass the entire body in Fitzgerald's zone therapy.

In 1968 two siblings, Dwight Byers and Eusebia Messenger, established the National Institute of Reflexology. By the early1970s the institute had grown and was renamed the International Institute of Reflexology.

In a typical reflexology treatment, the therapist and patient have a preliminary discussion prior to therapy, to enable the therapist to focus more accurately on the patient's specific complaints and to determine the appropriate pressure points for treatment.

A reflexology session involves pressure treatment that is most commonly administered in foot therapy sessions of approximately 40-45 minutes in duration. The foot therapy may be followed by a brief 15-minute hand therapy session. No artificial devices or special equipment are associated with this therapy. The human hand is the primary tool used in reflexology. The therapist applies controlled pressure with the thumb and forefinger, generally working toward the heel of the foot or the outer palm of the hand. Most reflexologists apply pressure with their thumbs bent; however, some also use simple implements, such as the eraser end of a pencil. Reflexology therapy is not massage, and it is not a substitute for medical treatment.

Reflexology is a complex system that identifies and addresses the mass of 7,000 nerve endings that are contained in the foot. Additional reflexology addresses the nerves that are located in the hand. This is a completely natural therapy that affords relief without the use of drugs. The Reflexology Association of America (RAA) formally discourages the use of oils or other preparations in performing this hands-on therapy.

Preparations

In order to realize maximum benefit from a reflexology session, the therapist as well as the patient should be situated so as to afford optimal comfort for both. Patients in general receive treatment in a reclining position, with the therapist positioned as necessary—to work on the bare feet, or alternately on the bare hands.

A reflexology patient removes both shoes and socks in order to receive treatment. No other preparation is involved. No prescription drugs, creams, oils, or lotions are used on the skin.

Precautions

Reflexology is extremely safe. It may even be self-administered in a limited form whenever desired. The qualified reflexologist offers a clear and open disclaimer that reflexology does not constitute medical treatment in any form, nor is reflexology given as a substitute for medical advice or treatment. The ultimate purpose of the therapy is to promote wellness; fundamentally it is a form of preventive therapy.

REFLEXOLOGY AND AROMATHERAPY BIBLE By Toni Austin

Chapter 1:

The Basics On Reflexology

Synopsis

This is a popular form of detecting and addressing any possible ailments, illnesses, or diseases the body may be undergoing. In ancient times this method was used to ensure that any possible negative problems in the body are arrested before it progresses to a point where it would be difficult to treat.

The Basics

Using reflexology to restore the equilibrium balance by means of the foot or hand is a rather strange but totally accurate. Many people have tried reflexology to address specific medical problems with overwhelmingly successful results.

The pressure sensors in the feet and hands are all connected to various parts of the body's systems. It functions like a network of intricate connections flowing from one to the other. By using reflexology, the experienced practitioner is able to pinpoint the cause of the problem and manipulate it through a succession of pressure points on the feet or palms of the hands. All these sensors work and respond to the sometimes light but mostly painful pressures on the feet and hands.

Other deviations but equally suitable forms of reflexology are walking on a pebble path, using foot massages that simulate reflexology movements, and using rollers. Surprisingly other simple tools like a golf ball can also be used as reflexology item though they are not as good as the original natural way of the thumb and finger.

Reflexology sessions ideally last for bout 30 – 45 minutes, as any longer might cause undue stress to the already pain heightened situation. The reflexologist uses pressure, stretches and movements to work thought the foot methodically. After which an assessment on the body condition may be given.

FAQ

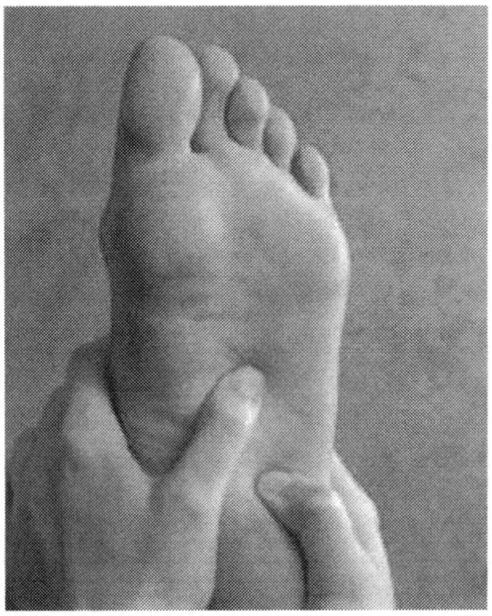

Is Reflexology safe?
Yes. Practitioners trained in the Original Ingham Method of Reflexology have the knowledge and skills to work with people of all ages, from newborn babies to the elderly, including the provision of professional reflexology during pregnancy, chemotherapy and palliative care.

Is Reflexology painful?
Reflexology can be extremely relaxing, however if there is a part of the body that is unbalanced, the corresponding reflex point may feel sore or tender whilst the practitioner works to rebalance the area. If at any time you find the treatment painful, please tell your Practitioner, as it is important that they work within your comfort-zone.

Is Reflexology ticklish?
No. The way in which a professional Reflexologist holds and works the feet is with a firm pressure which is not at all ticklish.

Chapter 2:

Reflexology Points And Areas

Synopsis

Ideally the chart on the subject on reflexology reflects the various pressure points and their corresponding parts of the different organs, glands, structures, and systems of the anatomy. These charts can also be looked upon as maps of the intricate workings of the human body.

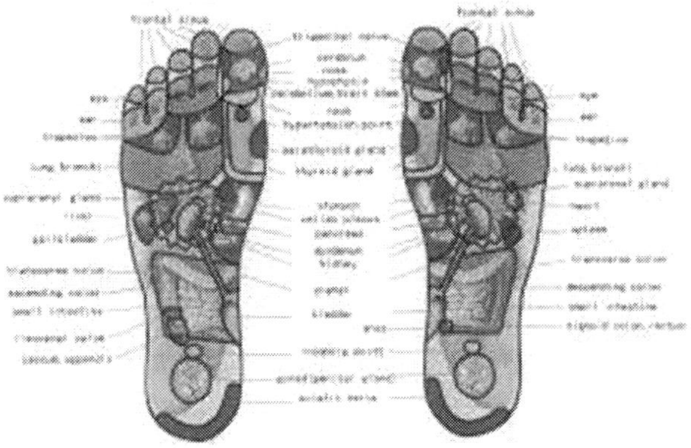

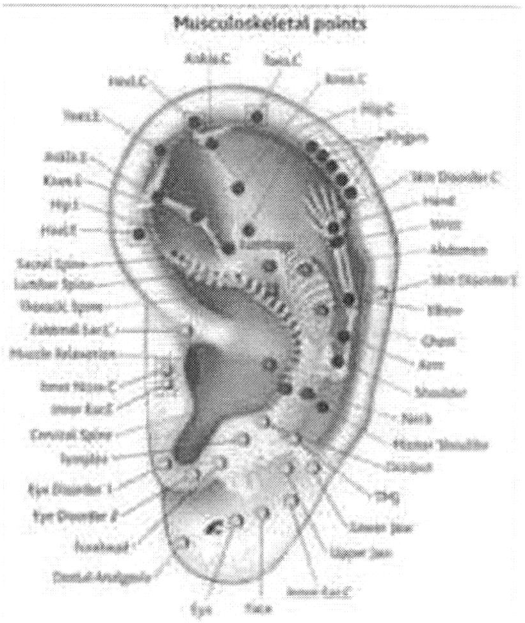
Musculoskeletal points
Hand
Abdomen
Elbow
Chest
Arm
Shoulder
Neck
Sacral Spine
Lumbar Spine
Muscle Relaxation
Cervical Spine
Eye Disorder 1
Eye Disorder 2
Lower Jaw
Upper Jaw
Dental Analgesia
Eye
Face

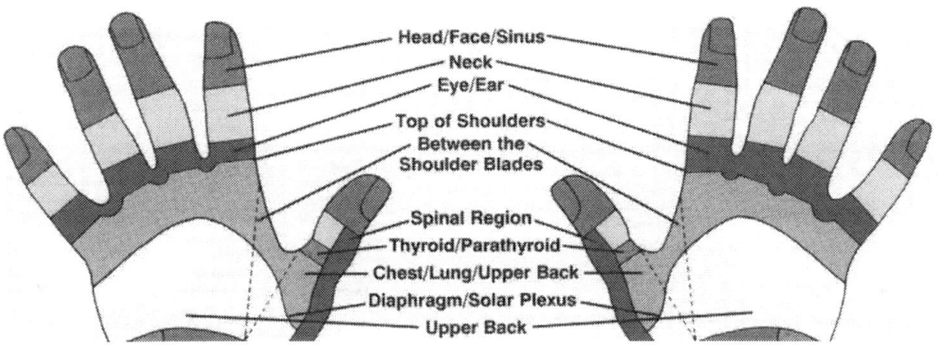
Head/Face/Sinus
Neck
Eye/Ear
Top of Shoulders
Between the Shoulder Blades
Spinal Region
Thyroid/Parathyroid
Chest/Lung/Upper Back
Diaphragm/Solar Plexus
Upper Back

The Areas

Though popularly accepted as a foot and hand, palm focused style of treatment; there are also instances of having the reflexology points in the ear area. Simply put, reflexology sessions strive to open up the stubble energy channels thus directing reflexology pressure points to stimulation mode.

The ear also has various pressure points which are connected to the autonomic functions of the heart and stomach. When addressed these pressure points seem to successfully invoke stronger autonomic responses in the cardiac and gastric systems when compared to the foot or palms. The ear lobes seem to contain master sensory points which affect the eyes, pineal and pituitary glands.

According to medical research there are 10 zones or meridians that are logistically located in the human body. For instance, when pressure is applied to the big toe the benefits are seen in the brain area. Likewise, when pressure is applied to the base of the foot, it treats the neck and throat ailments. Pressure on the ball of the foot puts the connection through to the lungs and heart. The foot arch when pressured affects the adrenals, kidneys, gastrointestinal track, and bladder. The middle of the foot when pressured affects the waistline, while the ankle bone affects sexual functions.

Being supposedly easy to detect these various pressure points and their connections for treatment is not reason enough to completely discontinue an ongoing medical treatment program. Even if reflexology is considered as an added complimenting factor, a doctor's opinion should always be sought, especially if the illness is serious.

Chapter 3:

Assisting The Cardiovascular System

Synopsis

Ideally when treating a particular illness, ailment or disease, it should not be the practice to only address the particular area affected but besides focusing on the affected area, the other parts of the body should also be looked into.

The Heart

When a reflexologist treats an individual this is the primary concern. The reflexologist not only focuses on the problem but also try to ensure all the other connecting factors are addressed too. Therefore, the individual facing cardiovascular problems should expect to be treated holistically as the art of reflexology demands.

As the cardiovascular system is made up of various corresponding part, which are the heart, arteries, veins, arterioles, venules and capillaries, it should be notes that the actual heart may not be the problem area. Its purpose is to carry all the nutrients and oxygen to the various parts of the body. When these are blocked for one reason or another then reflexology is a good first address.

Using reflexology to reestablish the optimum flow and circulation in the system is a good noninvasive way of treating the problem before it escalates to a more serious level.

Using reflexology, the heart reflexes are addressed as this organ is the instrument that pumps the blood thought-out the body. Then the kidneys are the next in line to be addressed.

The kidneys filter the blood constantly. The diaphragm and chest are also noted by the reflexologist because these reflexes would be worked to encourage relaxation in the chest cavity and promote deeper breathing.

Lastly the spinal area is also checked. Located on the inner edges of the feet the spine reflexes would be stimulated to promote communication through the nervous system.

Sometimes reflexology can also be used in the case of an actual heart attack, though it is not recommended if there is immediate medical response available.

Chapter 4:

Assisting Kidney Function

Synopsis

The kidneys in a human body have a vital part to play in maintaining the body at its optimum levels. This organ is responsible for eliminating all the waste and toxins from the body's circulatory system. When there is a buildup of all these negative elements the problems like renal failure may occur. Therefore, the cleansing method or condition the body should adopt to keep the negative buildups from occurring is by using reflexology.

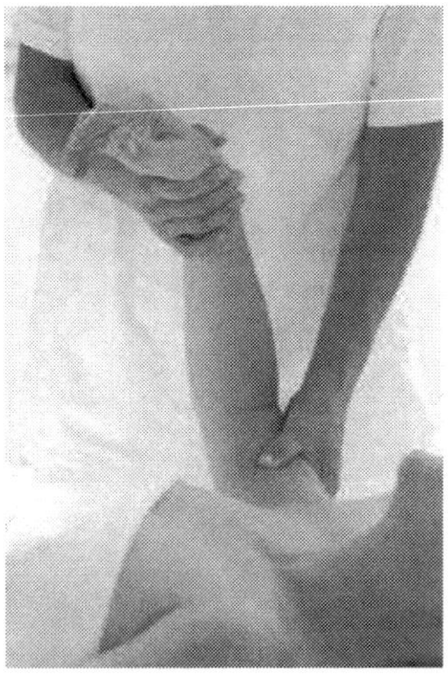

About The Toxins

Reflexology is a safe and proven method of addressing this, before it becomes a major problem for the body system. Making reflexology a good part of the health care regiment for an individual will help avoid any serious medical issues. Vectorial reflexology methods use very precise reflex points developed from the anatomy to eliminate any possible kidney problems.

When starting a reflexology session, the individual hand and feet should be easily accessible. The reflexology kidney zone is in the palm so by placing the individual's palm in the reflexologist hands and then applies pressure downwards between the index finger and the middle finger rub in deep movements.

After doing this for both palms, the reflexologist can now move on to the feet. By rubbing the thumbs down the foot to the bottom of the arch in-between the big toe and next to the other kidney zone is addressed. This area should be rubbed vigorously. All this is done for a reasonable period of time until the pain and discomfort disappears.

In using the reflexology exercise the intention is to create the ideal circumstance to assure the flow of energy is restored to its optimum levels again. These pressures should trigger the brain to discharge the negative direct current of regeneration in to the deficient are of the body. The intention is to help clear the interstitial space of congestive debris and bring the body to a more efficient cellular level.

Chapter 5:

Help With PMS

Synopsis

All women go through the time where a menstrual cycle is part of their lives. The lucky ones breeze through this time of the month comfortably while there are others who are not so lucky. They may experience symptoms like bloating, sleepless nights cravings mood swings and many others.

For Women

Reflexology has been known to be able to provide some form of relief to ease the discomfort brought on by the menstrual cycle or otherwise referred to as PMS.

Most people who sought this method to address the discomfort endured every month have been pleased with the results. The reflexologist will begin the session from a holistic point of view.

With this in mind, certain reflex parts will be emphasized as these areas are in direct correspondence to the body parts and organ being affected by the PMS condition.

The reflexologist will spend an extra amount of time on the kidney reflex are if the individual is complaining of bloating or of water retention symptoms.

The glands and organs responsible for regulating the hormones would be another area the reflexologist would focus on as this area generally affects the specific symptoms being experienced.

The areas that might be addressed are as listed below:

- The brain – this area is pin pointed because of the serotonin pathways
- Digestive system – also because of the serotonin element which can be found in

the intestinal walls

- Central nervous system – is another reflex area
- Endocrine system reflexes
- Relaxation techniques - using reflex points this area of tension is address as it does negatively affect the PMS cycle.

Reflexology should only be sought if the PMS symptoms are fairly mild or irritatingly uncomfortable.

If the PMS symptoms are of a more severe nature other medical sources should be consulted first.

As in all things disregarding proper medical treatment in favor of alternative style treatments should only be done with the knowledge and advice of a medical physician familiar with the individual's medical condition.

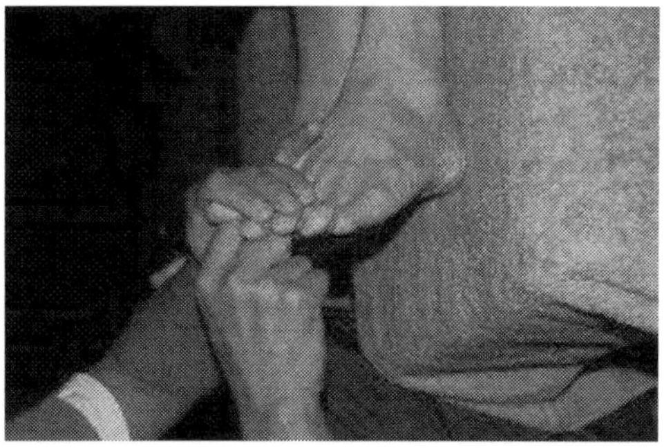

Chapter 6:

Bettering Quality Of Life For Cancer Patients

Synopsis

When an individual first discovers a dreaded disease like cancer is present in his or her body, the effects can be mentally devastating to say the least. Most people fall apart initially, for the lucky ones however, after absorbing the initial shock, they dive in and find out about the disease as much as possible and also all the relevant styles of medical or natural treatments that are available.

Some Relief

Reflexology has been one such discovery made. Many who use reflexology as a treatment that compliments the ongoing medical treatment have attested to being completely satisfied with the positive results. The commencement and incorporation of reflexology into the general treatment regiment, of course should only be done with a doctor's consent.

When the reflexology therapy is used to treat the patient, it is done with various intentions in mind. Some of these intentions are to provide comfort and peace of mind, to lessen the impact of side effects caused by the medical treatments, such as pain, anxiety, nausea, vomiting, fatigue, stress, depression, and fatigue. Other areas also to be addressed by reflexology are the improvements of the quality of life after chemotherapy, mood swings, quality of sleep, morale, and vital signs.

All cancer patients experience stress at various levels and at various intervals during the onset and treatment of the disease. As most negative medical conditions are somehow linked to causing more damage in the body system, reflexology can be used to correct the stress levels effectively. Reflexology is a gentle, effective tool used to assist in supporting and encouraging the patient to be in a better frame of mind and body.

By trying to create some sense of harmony in an already traumatic condition, reflexology works to play a positive role in creating a healing environment during and after the course of medical treatments.

Chapter 7:

Increasing Energy and Feelings Of Wellbeing

Synopsis

A good percentage of people today are very concerned with their health. This concern may lead them to take better care of the diet and prompt them to exercise more frequently and consistently.

However when there are medical problems, the first choice they usually make is to seek medical advice.

While this is of course a wise thing to do, some other alternatives may solve the problem better without the individual having to ingest foreign elements into the body to treat the condition.

The human body already comes with its own healing tools, but sometimes these tools just need that little help to ensure optimum successful results.

Step Up Your Vigor

One option to choose when experiencing mild medical problems is reflexology. Reflexology address the problem is a holistic manner and not just the problem itself.

All contributing factors, needs to be addressed, while detecting the root cause, and meting out the necessary pressures. As the toxins build up in our body systems, something should be done to address this condition before these said toxins begin to cause negative medical conditions. Reflexology helps to ensure all the body organs are working efficiently toward this goal.

In a reputably conducted reflexology session the individual can expect to benefit holistically because there are various aspects that are addressed. These include improving the general circulation in the body system, relieving pain, and stimulated the immune and nervous systems. Each body system is addressed individually with the intention of correcting any disorders that may be present.

The blood circulation system is addressed because it contributes to the wellbeing condition of the varicose veins, hemorrhoids, and high blood pressure. In the case of the digestive system, reflexology is sought to keep the following conditions under control or eliminate them all together; stomach upsets, stomach bloating, irritable bowel syndrome, colitis, diarrhea, and ulcers. The nervous system is for addressing any possible sleep disorders, depression, and lack of concentration or energy and memory loss.

Chapter 8:

Emotional Healing With Reflexology

Synopsis

The most common reason people seek out reflexology sessions is to ensure their stress levels are kept under control or eliminated altogether. This is because a stress free body is a healthy body.

Even if a foot massage is given without any real reflexology techniques, the receiver would be induced into a state of relaxation and peace. The more often an individual is able to have the peace and relaxation condition within the body system, the less stress levels are detected is any at all.

The Mind

Therefore, using reflexology to control emotions is beneficial to the overall health of an individual. As reflexology is used in general to support and encourage the body to right itself, it can be a major element in controlling the emotions that are the byproduct of various negative medical conditions.

Reflexology can be used to resolve the negative emotional states brought on by anger, grief, fear, guilt, stress, jealousy, and depression.

The negative energy is released out to the individual's system using the various pressure points related to addressing this particular issue. As the meridian system is the communicator between all the various organs any physiological systems the energy flow can be sustained at an optimum level using reflexology.

The effects of emotions have a direct impact on the health condition of the body as previously pointed out. The body consists of fluids like blood, lymph, urine, sweat, semen and cerebral-spinal fluid all of which are reflected in the feet and can be recognized by a trained and experienced reflexologist.

The fluids need to be in a constant flowing motion and when they are prevented from doing so, due to reasons like blockages then the problem cycle begins. Using reflexology to remove these blockages through the various pressure points is a good noninvasive excepted action.

Chapter 9:

Boosting Your Immune System

Synopsis

The human immune system is the first line of defense the body has for addressing potential negative elements. These elements may consist of viruses, diseases, illnesses and others. Understanding the immune system is very important to an individual's who intends to always stay healthy.

The Whole Body

Besides removing waste matter of the different forms, the immune system is responsible for protecting the body from external influences that are harmful to the body and facilitating the smooth flow of the interstitial fluids.

It also identifies all bacteria and pathogen cells and eliminates them. The immune system helps the various body parts to stay at optimum conditions in order to carry out all its particular functions successfully.

The smooth flow of the fluids can sometimes cause complications to the other functioning organs when there is a blockage. Reflexology can address this blockage of fluids properly and in a reasonable amount of time.

By listening to the bones, the reflexologist is able to tell if there are pulls in the connective tissues. If not remedied, these pulls, can affect the fluid flow patterns in the body.

Upon locating these pulls the reflexologist with then begin working on the foot, palm or ear areas to put pressure in specific points to try to relieve the area and relax the pulls until they reach their normal conditions.

Reflexology is also beneficial as a preventive measure for good health, with particular attention being paid to the immune system; the individual is able to keep the balance of the equilibrium thus aiding the body systems to work more efficiently. Regular treatments to address a specific problem, or just to ensure the body condition is in shape is a good habit to form.

If one's immune system is working efficiently then, there would be no need or a lesser need to visit the doctor so often. Also the immune system will be able to fight off any outside infections more successfully.

Chapter 10:

How To Do Reflexology

STEP BY STEP INSTRUCTIONS FOR FOOT REFLEXOLOGY!

Start now by learning the technique you will use;

Foot Reflexology Technique

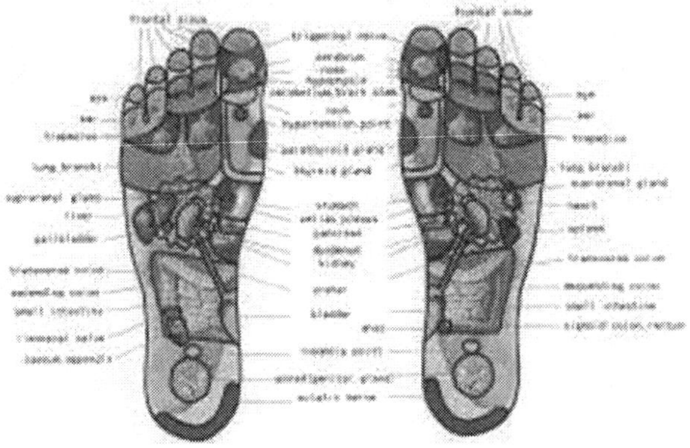

Thumb Walking

This is the most used technique for doing foot reflexology

It is easy, can be done for long periods of time without straining your hand and is extremely effective on the feet

Your thumb walks forward by itself simply by you bending and unbending the thumb.

Step 1.

Which part of the Thumb to use

1a. put your hands palm together in front of your face and look at the tops of your thumbs

1b. roll thumbs together at the top slightly so the nails are just touching

1c. feel the part of your thumbs where they are touching each other just on the inside at the top

This is the part of the thumb to use when thumb walking, the inside edge of the very top of your thumbs, (edge meaning that it is furthest away from the fingers of the same hand when the hand is put flat on a table)

Step 2.

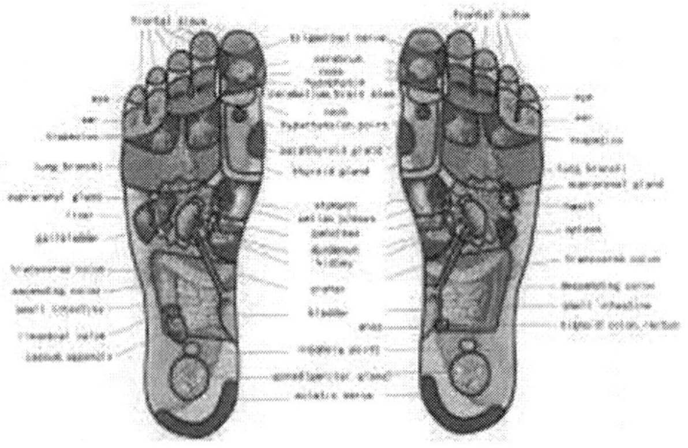

Thumb Walking Technique

2a. hold a pen with one hand (if you don't have a pen any similar surface is fine)

2b. with the other hand, put your thumb on the pen touching it with the part of the thumb described in the first step

2c. bend your thumb

2d. without moving anything else, simply straighten your thumb making sure that it stays in contact with the pen

You will notice two things

- your thumb crept slightly forward

- you are now able to apply a little bit of pressure with the part of your thumb that is touching the pen

2e. repeat; Bend, unbend, bend, unbend

Apply pressure at the unbend and creep forward in the bend.

Practice this technique slowly, it gets easier and faster with practice

It is easy learning foot reflexology techniques, pratically anything is a great surface to practice on; tables, chairs, TV remote controls... anything can be thumb walked!

This technique is used for the entire foot

Thumb walking allows a reflexologist to apply stimulating pressure to every single part of the foot, giving a thorough and relaxing treatment

How to do Reflexology on the Feet

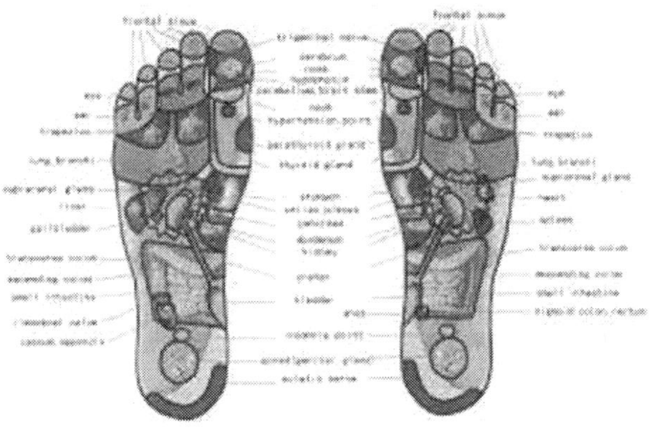

Begin every foot reflexology session on the right foot, do the whole foot, followed by the left.

Step 1.

Relaxation Exercises

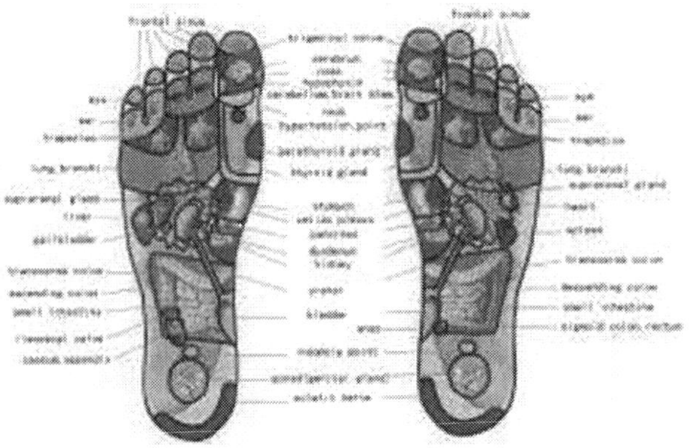

1a. massage the foot all over slowly but firmly to loosen it up, beginning at the toes moving down towards the heel, for about thirty seconds

1b. using both hands, hold on to the spine area with the palm of the hands- fingers on top of the foot and thumbs on bottom of the foot.

1c. slowly and gently twist/ wring the hands away from each other in order to gently twist the spine area on the foot. This is a relaxation exercise. Loosely wring one way and the other for about thirty seconds total

Step 2.

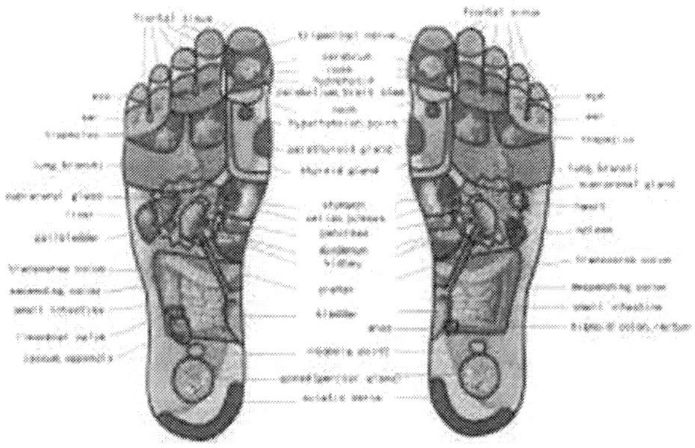

Thumb Walking the Spine

2a. thumb walk up the spine from the bottom of the heel to the tip of the big toe

2b. thumb walk down the spine from top of the tip of the big toe to the bottom of the heel

2c. thumb walk down the spine, but across-ways- from right to left for the entire length of the inside of the foot, see diagram below

Step 3.

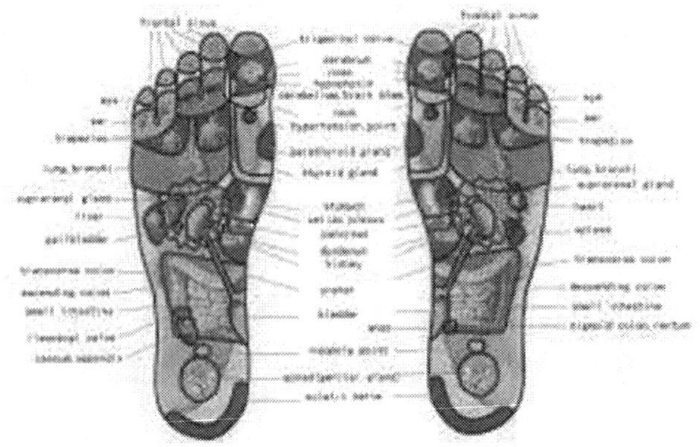

Rotate the Toes

Begin with big toe, continue toe by toe until the smallest end toe

3a. hold the toe firmly at the base of the toe, gently move in circular motions so that you are rotating and stretching the base joint that attaches the toe to the foot

3b. hold the toe just above the second joint and again move the joint in a large circular motion

3c. rotate the very top joint on the toe (the big toe only has two joints)

This foot reflexology step is great for relieving headaches as it relates to all of the bones in the skull, jaw... every bone in the head

When learning how to do reflexology remember the bones protecting our brain are fused together but are also separate bones, rotating the toes sends extra blood flow to their joints

Step 4.

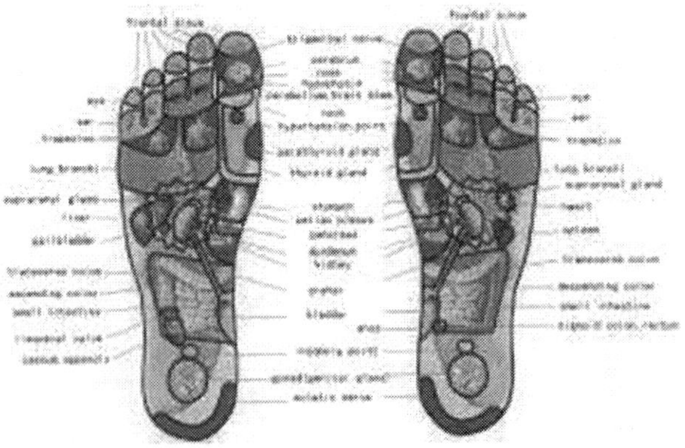

Stimulate Meridian Points on Toes

There are meridian points at the end of all the toes except the middle toe

See the diagram below for the exact points, they are easy to remember because they are pretty much under each toe nail!

4a. support the toe and use one finger to apply pressure on the meridian point in a circular motion - clockwise, then anti-clockwise, do each toe for ten seconds beginning with the big toe and finish with the little toe

Step 5.

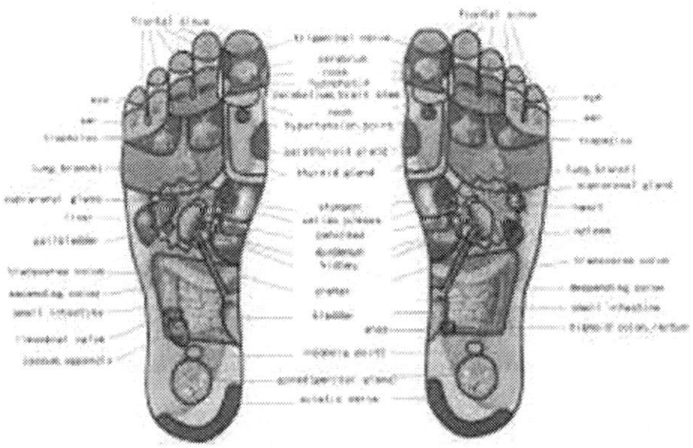

Thumb Walk the Toes

5a. thumb walk the toes in an upwards direction. Begin at the base and move upwards in a straight line to the tip.

Repeat on all sides of each toe, applying gentle but firm pressure. Begin with the big toe and finish with the little toe.

Some people like lots of pressure when thumb walking their feet, most people will not because it will stop the reflexology from being relaxing, and its supposed to be relaxing

Some peoples toes are extremely sensitive

The amount of pressure you use with any reflexology technique is relative to how much pressure the person is comfortable with, and so it is relaxing for them (although do be firm, too soft and you will tickle them!)

If there is pain in someones foot, take a break from doing reflexology on them for a while

Step 6.

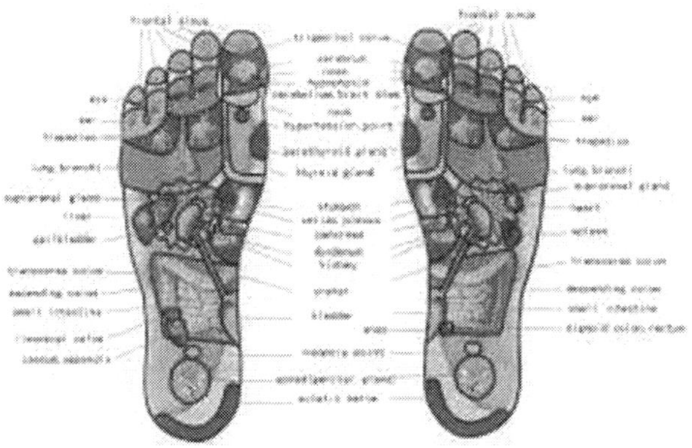

Thumb Walk Chest Area

The chest area is the ball of the foot

See exact area in foot reflexology diagram above

6a. gently thumb walk over the entire chest area in the upwards direction, then downwards and then on an angle

Step 7.

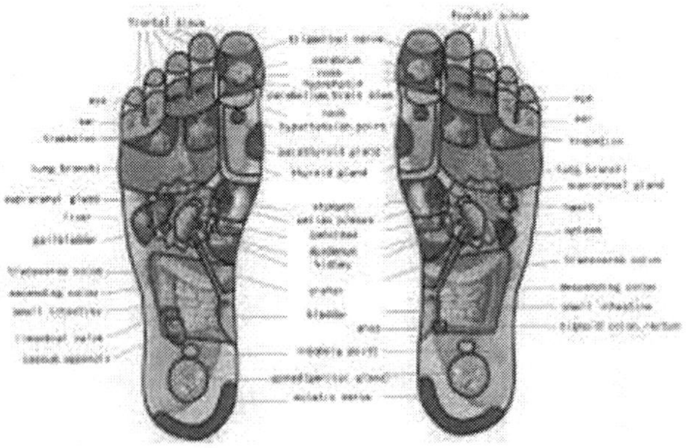

Thumb Walk Top and Back of Foot

This is a very sensitive area for most people.

7a. thumb walk from one side of the foot to the other side ie; from the toes to the ankle, for the entire top of the foot

7b. thumb walk from side to side- from right to left sides of the foot, for the entire top of the foot

Step 8.

Thumb Walk Liver/ Stomach area

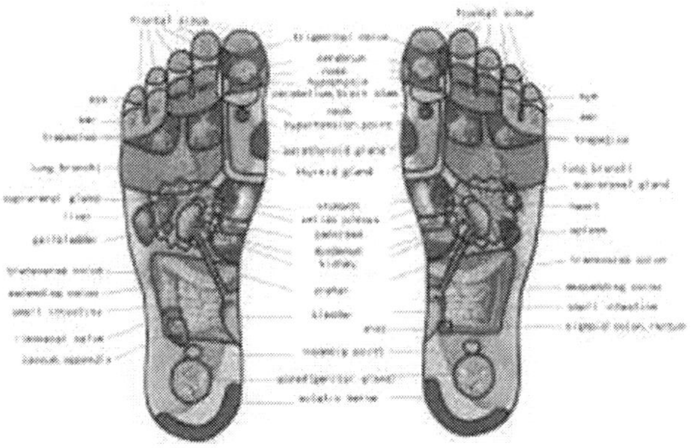

The waistline is the thinnest part of the bottom of the foot and may be further up or down and is in a different spot for everyone

Use the diagram at step six to locate the waistline

8a. thumb walk on an angle across the area between the chest area and above the waistline

8b. thumb walk on the opposite angle back across the area

This area contains the very important liver and stomach, depending on which foot you are working

Step 9.

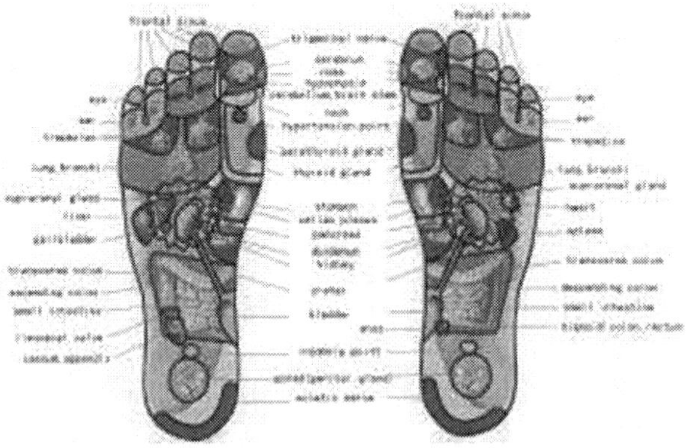

Thumb Walk Intestinal area

Use the diagram at step six to locate the waistline on the bottom of the foot

The large and small intestines are in this area

9a. thumb walk on an angle across the area between the waistline and the pelvic area

9b. thumb walk on the opposite angle back across the same area

For extra foot reflexology, check out the reflexology foot chart and see the direction that food moves through the intestines, and thumb walk in the same direction, the direction is different for the left and the right feet

Step 10.

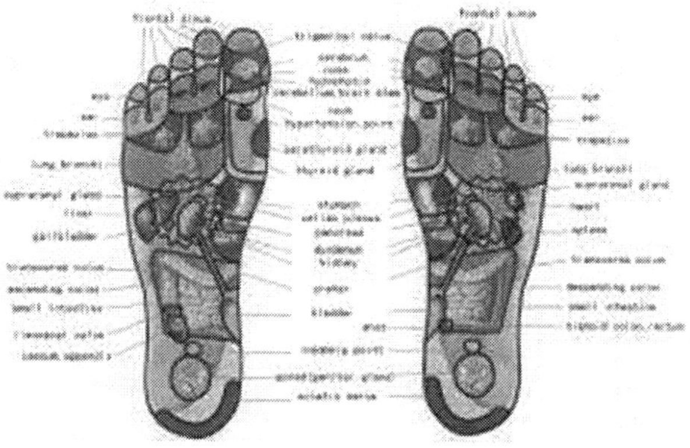

Thumb Walk Pelvic area

Use the diagram at step six to locate the pelvic area

This area relates to the Sciatic Nerve which runs up both legs

10. thumb walk from left to right over this area, go all the way up either side of the heel

10b. thumb walk the back of the heel

10c. finish reflexology with a gentle relaxing massage of the foot for one minute

Step 11.

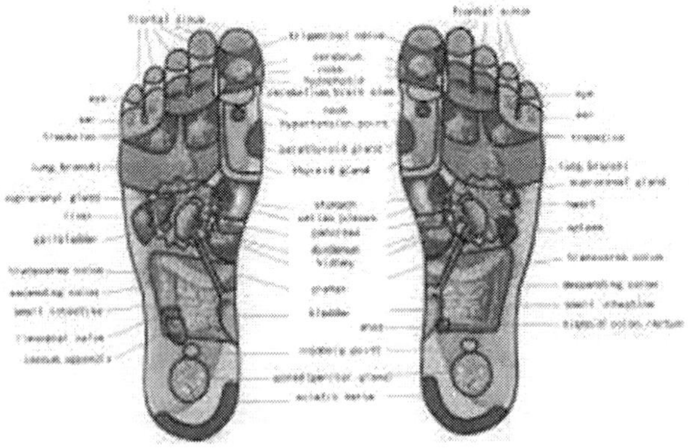

Repeat on Left Foot

11a. Go back to Step 1. and repeat each step on the left foot

CHAPTER 11

How To Do Self Reflexology, Find A Practitioner And Possible Side Effects

Synopsis

It is interesting to note that reflexology can be done as self help. In order to address certain specific problems a careful study of a reflexology chart must be done. Visiting a certified reflexologist for the initial consultation before embarking on the path on one's own would be better.

The Inside Info

Specific illnesses and problems are treated by targeting specific points. This can be located at the foot, palm of the hands and ears.

The easiest form of self reflexology is to follow these steps:

- While sitting comfortable bring the foot up and rest it over the opposite knee. Lace your fingers with your toes and rotate the foot at the ankle clockwise and then switch to anti-clockwise.
- Gently stretch the foot by pulling it upwards and back, all the while keeping the finger and toes laced.
- Place the ball of the foot or heel between both hands
- Placing the hands on either side of the foot gently but firmly apply pressure to each part starting with the toes, then alternate with a kneading motion.
- Forming knuckles press the first against the foot and then apply pressure going in an up and down motion.
- May finish off with a lotion rub to address any "missed" areas.

Wrapping Up

Though it may seem fairly easy to perform the reflexology moves on one's self there are some precautions that need to be taken and also some points that everyone needs to be weary off.

Certain conditions may not permit the reflexology to be done on the feet, perhaps due to the pain factor, then the exercise has to b=done on the palms of the hands.

When already ill, if reflexology is done on the feet, further toxins will be emitted into the body and this will cause a further deterioration of health.

If a fracture of broken bone condition has occurred it would be a serious folly to administer the reflexology style of treatment, as the pain involved will stress the individual further.

All in all, reflexology is safe, but always make sure to check with your doctor or reflexologist first.

BOOK 2

AROMATHERAPY

AROMATHERAPY

REFLEXOLOGY AND AROMATHERAPY BIBLE By Toni Austin

Copyright © 2016 by One Life Wellbeing
(OLW)
All rights reserved. No part of this publication may be reproduced, distributed, or transmitted in any form or by any means, including photocopying, recording, or other electronic or mechanical methods, without the prior written permission of the publisher, except in the case of brief quotations embodied in critical reviews and certain other non-commercial uses permitted by copyright law. For permission requests, write to the copyright holder at www.onelifewellbeing.com

REFLEXOLOGY AND AROMATHERAPY BIBLE By Toni Austin

LEGAL NOTICE

The Publisher has striven to be as accurate and complete as possible in the compilation of this book.

While all attempts have been made to verify information provided in this publication, the Publisher assumes no responsibility for errors, omissions, or contrary interpretation of the subject matter herein. Any perceived slights of specific persons, peoples, or organizations are unintentional.

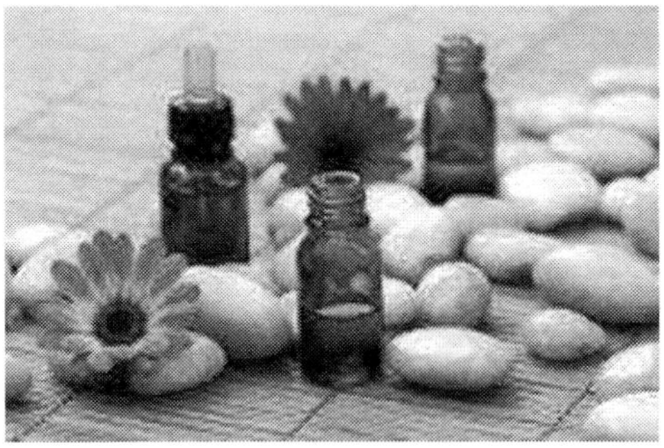

Foreword

Aromatherapy uses herbal oils to treat the mental, emotional and physical properties of an illness through the sense of smell. Herbs are fragrant and give off particular scents that each have properties thought to help heal certain illnesses. Aromatherapy is thought to be especially helpful to calm nerves and soothe anxiety.

Aromatherapy dates back to the uncharted mists of prehistoric times and has been used throughout history ever since. Incense is a form of aromatherapy that has been popular for thousands of years across many different cultures. Today, the use of aromatherapy is popular to help promote health and well-being and to reduce the effects of stress.

Aromatherapy works by releasing herb infused oils or liquids into the air. Essential oils may be placed onto a small cloth and then placed where the aroma can disperse throughout the area. Aromatherapy has become a popular and accepted method in the last several decades, and products are now widely available at local stores and supermarkets. Aromatherapy is used in many bath products and lotions. Examples of aromatherapy products include air fresheners or diffusers, as well as electric and battery powered products that spread the scent through the use of small fans.

Aromatherapy is a holistic approach to healing, taking into consideration the needs of the whole person. This takes into consideration your physical, mental and emotional states to help determine which essential oils are best suited for your particular situation. Aromatherapists mix essential oils together to create blends that are specific to your needs.

Your sense of smell is the only sense that actually has nerve receptors exposed outside the body. When a scent is detected special messages are transported to the limbic system inside the brain to be processed. The scent is identified there. This part of the brain also stores memories, which is why certain smells are often strongly associated with certain memories in your life. Blending essential oils together can form scents that are pleasant and relaxing, thus helping to reduce and eliminate stress and tension.

Essential oils are usually dissolved in either a water or oil base to blend together. The amounts used are small and do not cause any potential danger in these extremely low doses. These blends are often available as pre-made mixtures and are also able to be custom blended by an aromatherapist or by you at home.

Massage therapy uses aromatherapy to help in relaxation. Essential oils are used to massage the body. Besides the scent of the massage oil, small amounts of essential oils can also enter the body through the skin into the bloodstream. Again, these small doses are not considered harmful.

Although aromatherapy does not claim to cure any diseases, it is, nonetheless, responsible for helping soothe the body and mind in many ways. It can help improve your mood and general feelings of well-being. Specific combinations of essential oils can help create euphoric sensations in the brain. Aromatherapy can improve blood circulation and also improve lymphatic function when combined with massage therapy. Some soothing herbs are now used in common baby products to calm and help lessen the effects of colic and to help promote better sleep.

Herbs can be used in aromatherapy treatments in several ways. Essential oils are the easiest to use. These are made by distilling the plant material and mixing with a small amount of liquid or oil. Essential oils are concentrated and need to be diluted when used, and a few drops are all that is necessary when mixing with other oils. Essential oils can be used in baths, in lotions and perfumes and as inhalations. They are readily available at most health food or natural stores, as well as online. Do not put essential oils directly on the skin without first diluting them. These concentrations are strong and even safe herbs can cause irritations if not diluted. Be sure to dilute even more when using with young children.

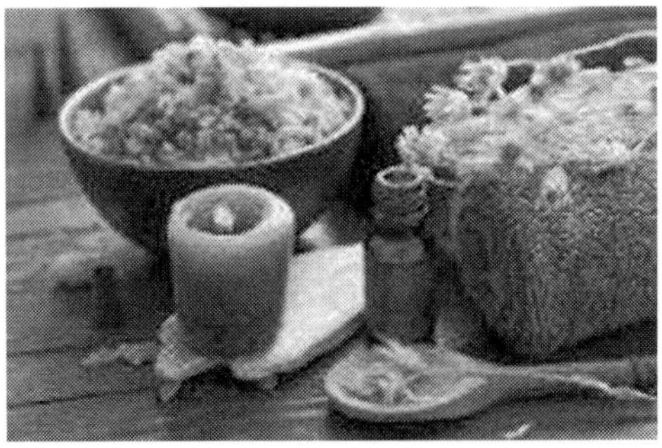

Chapter 1: Aromatherapy Basics

Occasionally divided into 3 distinctive areas of uses, aromatherapy has proven an effective resolution to a lot of problems. Aerial diffusion falls in the class for environmental fragrance or disinfection.

Direct inhalation is promoted to arrest assorted respiratory problems like respiratory disinfection, congestion, tautness in the chest cavity and a lot of others. Topical applications are chiefly for relaxing purposes like massages, baths, compresses and therapeutic skincare treatments.

In theory aromatherapy has been encouraged to be thought of as an alternate to more invasive sort of treatments. Besides being much more pleasant as a treatment choice it may occasionally even be touted as a prevention element to particular diseases.

At worst it may play a major role in relaxing the general state of an person and perhaps contribute in some way to the more successful part of recovery when combined with other more scientifically accepted techniques of treatment.

Nowadays there are a lot of avenues of treatment to explore before embarking on a certain sort suitable for the person. However it must always be noted that before making a choice, one must always try to be as well informed as possible.

The importance of understanding a certain topic, idea, or element is frequently overlooked in this busy world. To make matters worse it's frequently difficult to find the time to truly extensively explore certain topics. But with the use of assorted modern tools, this task may be not only fun but really informative also.

Most individuals nowadays think aromatherapy as just a different indulgent exercise the privileged few enjoy. But upon taking the time to delve deeper, one is likely to find a whole new prospect relating to the really diverse uses of aromatherapy.

Originating long before medical science made breakthroughs and discoveries; aromatherapy has had a lot of success stories to back it's a lot of fantastic attributes. The concept of utilizing aromatherapy to treat wounds and burns first came about when a scientist badly burned his hand while conducting an experiment and later it was utilized again successfully, as an antiseptic to treat the wounded soldiers during world war two.

Being the basis of natural materials, aromatherapy is less unsafe a technique to choose from, when deciding on the best fitted treatment for assorted illnesses. In essence aromatherapy is a treatment that could or might not help in the prevention of diseases by the use of essential oils.

When paired with the more conventional methods of treatments it has been found to produce impressive results, chiefly contributing as a calming ingredient to the equation.

Aromatherapy may have a positive affect on the limbic system through the olfactory system. It has likewise been known to have direct pharmacological effects. There have been studies done to prove the connection between the direct affects of use between aromatherapy coupled with other scientific techniques, but to date no absolute data has been forth coming.

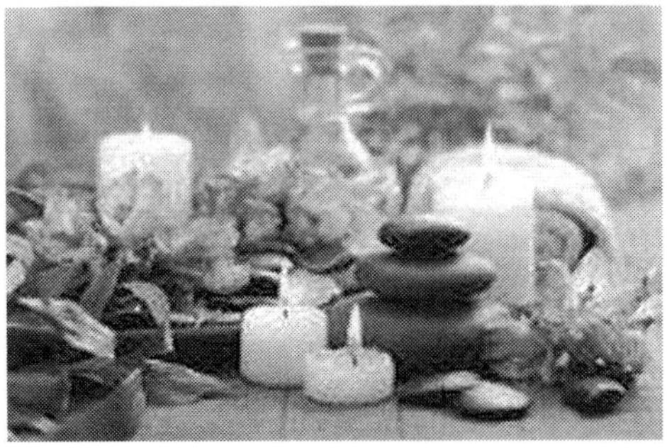

Chapter 2:

Tips for Getting Started

Synopsis

Here are some good tips for getting started with aromatherapy and essential oils.

For The Novice

Don't purchase perfume oils thinking they're the same thing as essential oils. Perfume oils don't offer the healing benefits of essential oils. Even if you merely intend on using aromatherapy in your life for the out-and-out enjoyment of the aroma, essential oils that are breathed in may provide therapeutic advantages. These advantages don't happen with the utilization of perfume oils.

Don't purchase essential oils with rubber glass dropper tops. Essential oils are really concentrated and will turn the rubber to a gum therefore ruining the oil.

Read as much as you are able to on Aromatherapy. It's really simple to get going with Aromatherapy, however there are safety concerns that you need to be aware of. You're wise to read even further on the significant subject of essential oil safety.

Be choosy of where you buy your essential oils. The quality varies widely from company to company. In addition, a few companies might falsely claim that their oils are pure when they aren't.

Learn to equate apples to apples if shopping for oils. Anise, lilac, bay laurel, cedar, and eucalyptus are examples of the basic names of plants utilized to make essential oils. There, however, are assorted varieties of each of these plants. To differential these varieties, the botanical name is utilized to tell them apart. For example, two assorted oils are referred to as "bay laurel essential oil," yet they come from 2 assorted plants. The attributes and aroma of each oil do differ as does the basic cost between the two. It, consequently, is crucial to pay attention to the botanical name.

It's likewise helpful to note the native land for the oil. Most great essential oil sellers will promptly supply the botanical names and native land for the oils that they sell. When comparing one company's oils with another's, likewise pay attention to if the oils are organic, wild-crafted or ethically produced.

It's wise not to buy oils from vendors at street fairs, craft shows, or other limited-time events. A few vendors understand novices have no recourse against them later. This isn't to say that there are not extremely reputable sellers at these events; however this is a precaution for novices who aren't able to dependably gauge quality.

Buying oils from reputable mail-order companies might result in obtaining higher quality oils at lower expense than buying oils from a generic local health food place of business. Again, there's a wide variance in the quality of oils from company to company and store to store.

Store your oils in dark glass (amber or cobalt blue) and in a cool, dark place. Bare wooden boxes may be bought at craft stores. These boxes let me to move my oils from assorted areas of the house easily. Wooden diskette holders can likewise serve this purpose well.

Pay special care and attention to all safety data on all essential oils that you use. This is even more crucial if you have any medical condition or are pregnant.

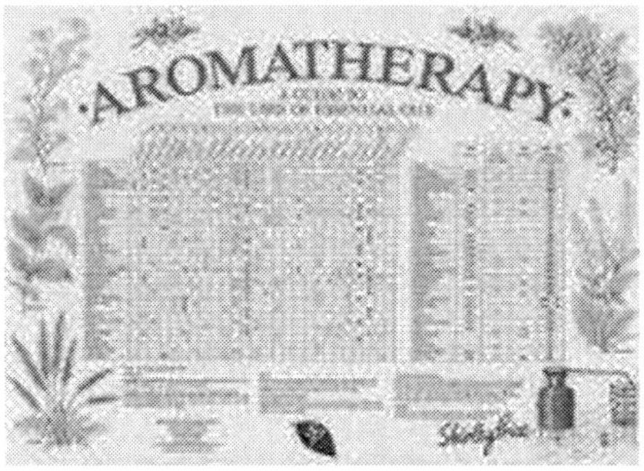

Chapter 3:

Choosing How To Use It

What Can Be Done

Most essential oils today are so commercialized that it might not always be as genuine as declared on the labels. Cautious examination of the label contents has to be checked and rechecked before an investment is made.

A few labels may be quite deceiving in their supposed capabilities. The condition and sort of packing of the essential oils is likewise a really crucial feature that ought to be considered. Ideally there shouldn't be any cracks or broken seals as this will impart contamination of the purity levels of the oils.

Besides all this, the additional crucial fact to consider is getting the fullest results through the technique and choice of essential oils.

Meaning a few essential oils work better when utilized the correct way and the most beneficial results are assured if the suggested way isn't taken for granted but stuck to carefully.

The technique of aspiration is utilized to treat particular ailments like sinuses, headaches, colds, chest congestions and additional like conditions. This technique is far more effective and faster than taking orally or direct application on the skin.

Spraying a variety of essential oils and distilled water is another technique utilized to produce a calming and relaxing ambiance. This technique has proved to be advantageous when treating nervousness, depression, stress and additional pressurizing conditions.

A few conditions demand direct applications. But as most aromatherapy massage session are executed with direct skin contact, the concentration of the essential oils needs to be thought of before beginning. Reason being that these essential oils may cause an allergic reaction to the person.

Utilizing essential oils that contain the Helichrysum ingredient has been demonstrated to be advantageous when repairing damaged skin.

Its strong anti-inflammatory and concentration of regenerative diketones is what makes it an extremely regarded compound in addressing damaged skin. The pleasing earthy scent it emits is likewise therapeutic.

Additional essential oils that are likewise known for their healing attributes for skin conditions are lilac, sage and rosemary. Sage is especially effective in healing old scars and stretch marks but ought to only be utilized is small amounts because of the Thujone content which may be toxic.
Utilizing aromatherapy to care for wounds is likewise widely practiced. This is because of the antiseptic components that particular essential oils contain. Tea tree essential oil is usually utilized to treat wound till the wound is completely sealed, after which this oil is no longer required.
A few aromatherapy treatments are likewise utilized when the desire for sound, younger looking skin is sought. These essential oils are soaked up into the skin and in turn provide the skin with all the crucial nutrients required for the healthy look and condition.
Aromatherapy is likewise utilized in additional products besides skin care. Products like bath salts, shower gels, shampoos, body lotions.
This style of utilizing aromatherapy is fantastic for producing the desired effects of sweet-scented and relaxing moods. Likewise aromatherapy in this form is mild and non-menacing as it is not in its purest form.
Aromatherapy may likewise assist in relieving restlessness and irritability. Essential oils like lilac may have calming effects on the mental turmoil state and works by promoting the senses to slow down and simulates peace.

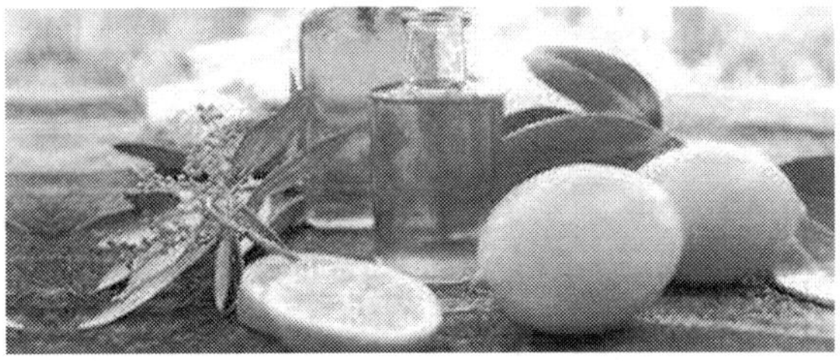

Chapter 4:

Recipes

Making your own personal essential oil blends is among the most satisfying facets of aromatherapy. Blends may be produced for the sheer aromatic pleasure of the blend and are suited for personal or room fragrance.

Essential oil blends may also be produced for particular therapeutic purposes like alleviating aching muscles, minimizing the occurrence of acne, reducing winter "blahs" etc...

Recipes

Aromatherapy Bath Oil Recipe

- 2 ounces carrier oil like Jojoba
- 20 drops lilac Essential Oil or 15-20 drops of your own blend of essential oils (make sure they are EOs that are not known to be skin irritants)

Instructions: Blend the oils together and store in a glass bottle. The formula could be doubled or tripled.

To Use: don't utilize all 2 ounces of bath oil in one bath. After you've drawn your bathwater, add about 1/4 ounce (7-8ml) of the bath oil blend to your water.

Mix well to ensure that the blend has scattered well in the tub and get on in. It's best to add the bath oil right before getting in the tub rather than while the water is running so that the essential oils don't vaporize before you get into the tub.

Utilizing this bath oil blend is safer than putting in pure EOs directly to the bath water. This is because pure essential oils added to bathwater may settle in one spot on your skin and cause aggravation.

Aromatherapy Bath Salts Recipe

- 3 C salt. Suggested salt types: Sea Salt, Dead Sea Salt, Himalayan Pink Salt, Epsom salt, or a combining of these salts. Salts commonly come in various grain sizes. Blending multiple grain sizes may make your salts more visually appealing. While chunkier salts frequently look prettier, bigger salts do take longer to break up in the tub and may be a little painful if you step or sit on some chunks that haven't totally broke up.

- 15-24 drops of your decided essential oil or essential oil blend. Make sure and take heed in the safety data for the oil(s) you decide to utilize.
- Optional: 1 TB JoJoba, Fractionated Coconut Oil or additional carrier oil for moisturization.

Instructions:
Place the salt mixture into a bowl. If you've decided to include the optional oil inside your salt recipe, add it to the plain salts and blend well with a spoon or fork. And then, add the drops of your decided essential oils.
Once again, mix really well. Add the mixture to a pretty jar, salt tube, or container that has a tightly fitting lid. Salts that are kept in a container that's not air tight will lose their scent more quickly.
After a day, you might wish to mix well again to ensure that the oils are well blended.
To Color to Your Salts:
For the rawest bath salt recipe, leave your bath salts undyed. Particular exotic salts including Hawaiian Red Sea Salt and Black Sea Pink Salt are by nature colorful. Try blending these salts with Dead Sea or plain sea salt for a flecked effect.
If you would like to add color to your salts, FD&C liquid dye or mica powder may be imparted before you add the essential oils. When putting in FD&C grade liquid dye, make sure to add only a drop at a time and mix well.
When adding mica powder, only add a flyspeck amount (1/16-1/8 a teaspoon is commonly sufficient) and mix really well. Utilizing too much dye or mica powder may discolor the water and discolor skin, so be really careful.
Leave bath salts at a soft pastel color. It's likewise crucial that you make certain that you're using skin-safe colorants and that the user of your bath salt blend doesn't have any allergic reaction or sensitizations to the colorant that you've selected.
To utilize:
Add 1/2-1 cup of the salts to running tub water. Blend well to ensure that the salt has scattered well in the tub prior to entering. To keep the essential oils from vaporizing too quickly, you may add the bath salts right before getting in the tub rather than while the water is running.

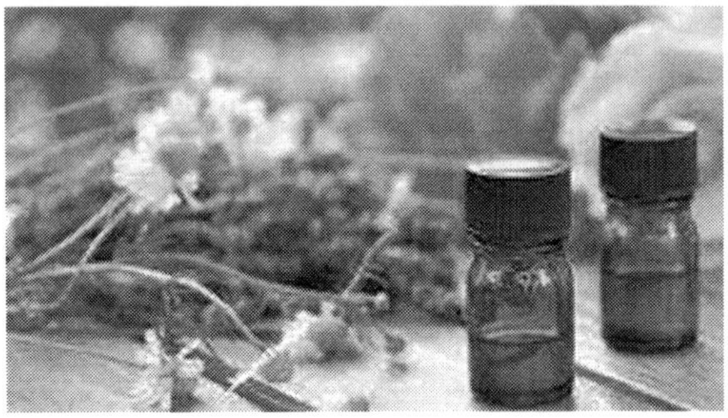

Chapter 5:

For What Ails You

Synopsis

The popular notion that most illnesses and diseases are in some manner linked to stress, anxiety and lack of proper daily nutrition has its virtues.

Regrettably some illnesses and diseases need to reach a critical stage before it becomes visible or is detected. To prevent all this, one is encouraged, although unrealistically, to keep all negative aspects in life in check or eliminate them all in all.

Aromatherapy may helpfully contribute to this end. Chiefly known for its calming properties, aromatherapy techniques advocate the utilization of various essential oils to comfort the mind and body.

Besides this long list there are other conditions that may be successfully addressed with the use of aromatherapy elements.

Some Healing

Below are just a few examples of the capabilities and merits of using aromatherapy:

Many herbs are used, and here are some of the most common herbs that are used in essential oils for aromatherapy.

Lavender - Lavender helps relieve tired muscles and can actually reduce muscle spasms. It is a very safe herb and is often used in many items, especially in baby products because of its gentle nature. There are relatively no side effects from using lavender. It is often used to calm anxiety and helps in eliminating insomnia. A diluted version is often used in a spray that can be used on beds and pillows to promote sleep. It is often used in small pillows that can be heated in the microwave and then applied onto the neck and back muscles to help relax them. Lavender blends well with most other herbs, making it a perfect choice for many herbal mixtures.

Bergamot - Bergamot is very uplifting. It is often used to help depression or mood swings. It is also helpful in eliminating insomnia and is said to help stop nightmares from occurring. It is a mild herb and is unlikely to cause any ill effects. It mixes well with most other herbs, including lavender, cedarwood, rosemary, geranium and lemongrass.

Tea Tree - Tea tree oil is an herb that is often used in topical mixtures to help fight bacterial infections. Used in aromatherapy, tea tree is said to help promote energy and helps relieve anxiety. It is also used to help aid in poor concentration. Another mild herb, tea tree is not associated with any known side effects and is safe to use. It mixes well with eucalyptus, bergamot, lavender and peppermint.

Neroli - Neroli is often used to help control the signs of stress and anxiety. Long used as a remedy, neroli is known to help those with exhaustion feel better and more relaxed. It helps with panic disorders and is said to calm fears, insomnia, and moodiness. It was used for many years as a treatment for grieving widows as it helps calm and soothe the mind. Neroli is a mild and safe treatment, and it blends well with most other herbs, including ylang-ylang, jasmine, melissa and peppermint.

Melissa - Melissa is known for its antiseptic properties when used on the skin. In aromatherapy, melissa is known to ease panic attacks. It is also used to help those who are overcoming addictions with alcohol or tobacco, as it helps alleviate those cravings.

Melissa helps encourage calmness and brings serenity to you, and helps stop fear and depression. It mixes well with most other herbs, especially jasmine, neroli, geranium, and chamomile. Melissa in aromatherapy is mild, but when used on the skin it can cause irritation for those with sensitive skin. Test a small spot on the skin prior to use.

Frankincense - Frankincense has been used for thousands of years and has strong religious associations to the Bible. It is a popular herb used to help restore confidence and calm. It helps calm fears and paranoia, as well as nightmares. It helps restore balance to those who have signs of emotional exhaustion. It is mild and is unlikely to cause any adverse reactions, and mixes well with most other herbs, including ylang-ylang, myrrh, neroli, melissa, cedarwood, rosemary and lavender.

Juniper - Juniper is commonly grown in the United States as well as Europe. The berries are very pungent and are used in the making of gin. Juniper is used to clear and stimulate the mind, and is said to prevent worry and unpleasant memories. It can renew enthusiasm and give you a new zest for life. It is safe as an aromatic; however, you should use caution when ingesting it if you have any kidney disease. Juniper blends well with most other herbs such as lavender, frankincense, tea tree and jasmine.

Whether improving mood or overall health, a winning strategy begins with stress reduction. And for the physical body that interprets stress as pain, these five essential oils know just where it hurts:

Lavender

Easily the most popular of all essential oils, lavender is known as the "universal oil." With its calming, earthy, lightly sweet and freshly floral scent, it is widely beloved for its relaxing and balancing effects on both the physical and emotional bodies. It may also be used as a pain reliever for muscles and joints, or as an antiseptic on minor cuts, burns, bug bites and stings.

Frankincense

With its comforting warm, exotic aroma, Frankincense's most common use is stress relief; however, it may also be applied topically to the skin to rejuvenate cells and repair scar tissue, or used to calm certain respiratory conditions such as asthma, coughing and bronchitis.

Rose

Another highly versatile essential oil, this one may be even more costly than most, due to its labor-intensive extraction process, which requires 60,000 roses for every one ounce of rose oil. In addition to providing relief from both stress and depression, the many uses of rose oil include the treatment of eczema and menopausal symptoms.

Chamomile

Though both the Roman and German types of chamomile essential oils are well suited for calming the nerves and supporting digestive health, there are some important differences between the two. Where the Roman variety is superior in addressing mental anxiety, paranoia and hostility, the German variety excels more in the treatment of irritated skin.

Vanilla

If the pure scent of warm vanilla makes you feel right at home, some aromatherapists say it is because vanilla is the closest in fragrance and flavor to mothers' milk. With the ability to both soothe in tranquil relaxation and stimulate mental clarity, this rich aroma can vary in its therapeutic effects. Vanilla essential oil has also proven effective in relieving upset stomachs and reducing cravings for sweets.

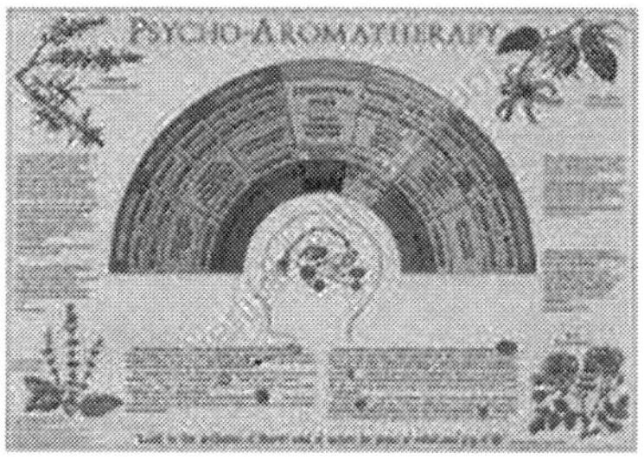

9 BEST ESSENTIAL OILS FOR SLEEP

1. VALARIAL

calming to the nervous system and helps with restlessness

2. VALOR

balances the nervous system and helps strengthen the body and mind; increases feelings of strength, courage, and self-esteem; Can also be useful for snoring.

3. VETIVER

relaxes the nervous system and helps with overstimulation

4. ROMAN CHAMOMILE

has a warm, sweet, herbaceous scent that is relaxing and calming for both mind and body. Its gentleness makes it especially valuable for restless children.

5. LAVENDER

very calming and can be good for anxious feelings

6. PEACE AND CALMING

promotes relaxation and a deep sense of peace and emotional well-being: helps release negative emotions: wonderful for children

7. CEDARWOOD

relaxing and soothing; allows the brain to stop processing

8. STRESSAWAY

brings feelings of peace and tranquility; helps to relive daily stress and anxious feelings; promotes relaxation; restores equilibrium

9. ORANGE

lifts the spirit while providing a calming influence on the body; brings peace and happiness to the mind. It is rich in the powerful antioxidant d-limonene and aids in maintaining normal cellular regeneration.

SLEEPY TIME ESSENTIAL OIL BLEND

Ingredients:

12 drops Orange
8 drops Lavender
4 drops Cedarwood
3 drops Valerian
2 drops Roman Chamomile
Directions:
Mix oils in a clean, glass essential oil bottle. Use in diffuser, inhale, topically, or in a warm bath mixed with epsom salt.

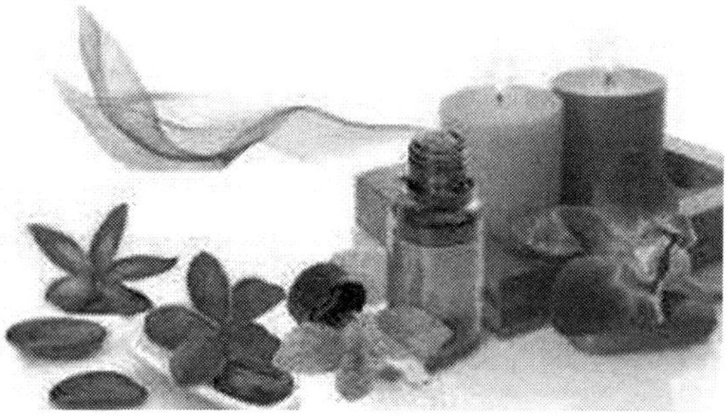

Here are some additional conditions where aromatherapy can be extremely helpful

Acne - lavender oil or tea tree oil to be used directly on the affected area. For milder cases, utilizing a body bath lotion with these properties is advocated.
Anemia - a concoction of tincture from the yellow dock root or an extract of dandelion leaf or even eating dandelion greens as a salad.
Anxiety - chamomile, California poppy, passion flower, lemon balm
Asthma - ginkgo biloba, mullein oil, a Chinese herb called shuan huang lian
Bee sting - urtica urens , cantharis, lavender and vegetable oil mixed
Body odor - alfalfa contains chlorophyll.
Cold - eucalyptus oil in boiling water and inhaled. Gargle with a mixture of tea tree oil
Cholesterol - chicory root, ginger
Constipation - aloe vera juice, ginger tea
Hair loss - saw palmetto, arnica, jojoba oil
Headaches - chamomile relaxes, ginkgo biloba improves blood circulation
Dandruff - flaxseed oil, primrose oil or salmon oil. Rinsing hair in chaparral or thyme
Diabetes - huckleberry, tea made from most beans
Diarrhea - blackberry tea, wild oregano
Eczema - chickweed added to bath, stinging nettle, hazel ointment
Indigestion - gentian root for better digestion, ginger, peppermint
Nausea and vomiting - catnip leaves, chamomile flowers

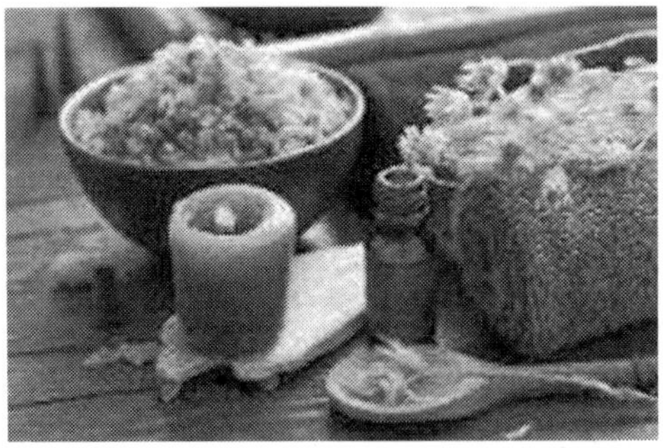

Chapter 6:

For Romance

For Love

While the words sensuality and sensual are frequently misapplied, a sensual person is one that has an intense awareness and admiration of the subtle changes that impact each of the senses.

Such a person tends to value creativeness and tends to have an exceptional interest in activities that capitalize on the senses. Such activities include assorted forms of music, culinary innovations, the visual arts, aromatics and assorted forms of physical touch including those that permit the physical manifestation of love and desire.

Aromatherapy, natural botanicals and natural fragrance all tease our sense of smell. They play an important role within romance, love and intimacy.

Fragranced room sprays, body mists, bath oils, rub down oils, and additional natural aromatics may heighten a romantic evening or impart variety and intrigue to your union.

Including aromatherapy and natural aromatics in your plans for romance won't suddenly make a stubborn, unromantic and impassionate person get more loving or sensual, however it may enhance his/her total mood, and make a romantic evening much more sensual. A room finely fragranced with a fresh and exotic aroma may help melt away worries and lift up the spirit while setting the stage for the evening's plans.

Planning beforehand for special dates, evenings or additional times may help ensure a quiet (or interesting!), beautiful occasion. Assigning special thought into all the aspects of a beautiful evening will make your mate feel special and prized, and will make the event unforgettable in his/her mind.

A great deal, all the same, may also be said about the advantages and wonders of spontaneous times. Impromptu moments may rule out including a few aromatic practices; however, it's likewise possible to plan ahead. A lovely selection of natural aromatics may be bought or prepared beforehand so that you have them on hand for if the mood strikes.

An aphrodisiac is broadly defined as a substance that enhances or arouses passion and sexual arousal. Substances, including essential oils, that are thought of as aphrodisiacs are substances that may help disperse the physical, psychological or emotional ailments that might interfere with physical attraction or arousal.

Wrapping Up

Aromatherapy or differently called essential oil therapy is a natural, gentle and non-invasive way of addressing a certain disorder. It may also be utilized to compliment an existing treatment regimen.
Occasionally aromatherapy may also be utilized as the only treatment.

Because of its soothing effect, aromatherapy may be utilized in treating ailments that require the patient to be in a non-trying state of body and mind. A few researchers have discovered that by inhaling particular scents, a patient may immediately bring in check the stressful nature of the predicament which contributes to the disease or illness suffered.

QUICK REFERENCE CHARTS

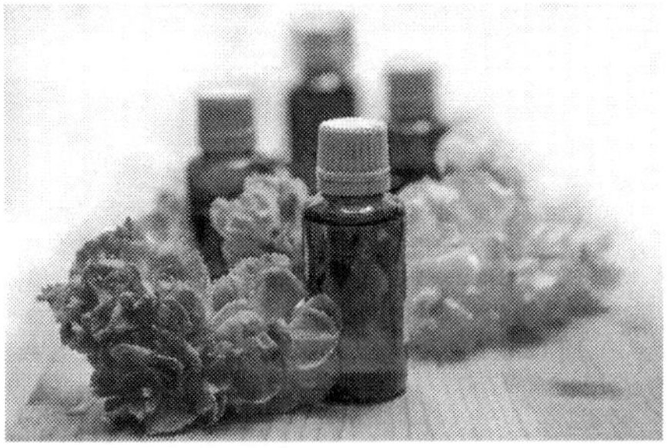

Aromatherapy Essential Oil Reference Charts

Oil	Properties	Uses	Precautions	Part of Plant Used
Cedarwood (Cedrus Atlantica)	antiseptic astringent energizing stimulant	stress tension deodorant insect repellent		wood
Chamomile (Matricaria chamomilla)	anti- inflammatory antidepressant disinfectant soothing diuretic	anxiety depression irritability stress		flowers
Citronella (Cymbopogon nardus)	energizing stimulating soothing	insect repellent		all parts

Clary Sage (Salvia sclarea)	antispasmodic calming relaxing soothing tonic warming	moodiness panic restlessness stress tension	do not use during pregnancy	flowering tops
Eucalyptus (Eucalyptus globulus)	antiseptic antiviral bactericidal decongestant expectorant stimulating	frustration anger stress tension depression		leaves & twigs
Frankincense (Buswellia thurifera)	calming grounding, toning	aging skin disturbed sleep fear grief stress vulnerability		resin
Grapefruit (Citrus paradisi)	energizing freshening, tonic	air freshener cellulite depression lethargy seasonal affective disorder (SAD) congestion	sun sensitivity	peel of fruit
Jasmine (absolute) (Jasmineum officinale)	aphrodisiac antidepressant energizing soothing uplifting	anxiety apathy depression nervous tension shyness	do not use during pregnancy	flowers
Juniper (Juniperus communis)	antimicrobial antiseptic astringent energizing	confusion exhaustion emotional distress	do not use during pregnancy	berries

Lavender (Lavandula officinalis)	analgesic antidepressant antimicrobial antiseptic bactericidal balancing calming soothing anti-inflammatory	anxiety fear insomnia hysteria depression panic restlessness		flowering tops
Lemon (Citrus limonum)	anti-infectious antiseptic bactericidal uplifting	refreshing nervous conditions	sun sensitivity	rind of fruit
Orange (Citrus aurantium)	cleansing antidepressant astringent calming mildly sedative tonic	anxiety depression insomnia	sun sensitivity	rind of fruit
Patchouli (Pogostemon patchouli)	antidepressant anti-inflammatory antiseptic aphrodisiac astringent calming soothing insecticidal	earth grounding anxiety depression stress acne athlete's foot dandruff		leaves
Peppermint (Mentha piperata)	decongestant energizing stimulating	centering focus grounding		leaves
Rose (Rosa damascena)	antidepressant aphrodisiac antiseptic calming centering	anxiety depression hopelessness insecurity	do not use during pregnancy	flowers

Rosemary (Rosmarius officinalis)	analgesic antiseptic energizing stimulating	focus concentration indecision procrastination hangover head aches muscular tension	do not use during pregnancy or if epileptic	leaves & flowering tips
Sandalwood (Santalum album)	antiseptic aphrodisiac astringent calming sedative soothing	apprehension depression shyness timidity		wood
Tea Tree (Melaleuca alternifolia)	antifungal anti-infectious antimicrobial antiseptic decongestant antiviral disinfectant energizing stimulant	athlete's foot acne infections psoriasis dandruff sinusitis		

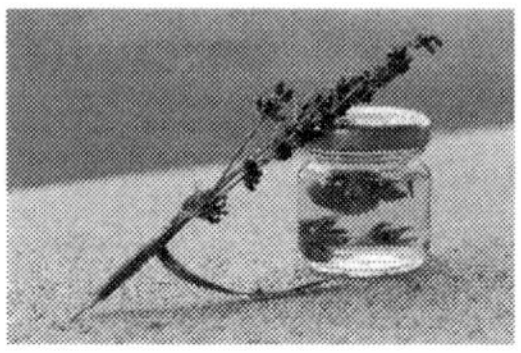

Dosage Reference Chart

Quick Reference Chart of Dosages and Directions for Treatment

Applications Essential Oil Drop Dosage

Aromatic Wrap Soak sheeting in10-15 drops and hand-hot water **Bathe** 4 drops in a small dish of cold boiled water **Bath** 6-8 drops in bath filled with warm water

Body Scrub Massage blend applied to body brush

Compress 6-8 drops in cold or warm water

Friction Rub 50/50 dilution in Lavender or base oil

Hand Friction Rub 2 drops neat to palm. rub to heat. Cup hands , inhale deeply

Hydrosol Spray 5 drops to 20mls of hydrosol spray (floral water)

Gargle 1-2 drops in a glass cold boiled water

Steam inhalation 2-3 drops in bowl of steaming water

Massage Ratio of one drop to 2ml base oil as a general guide

Neat	1 drop direct topical application to skin
Paper Funnel Inhalation	2-3 drops in base of paper towel, rolled into a cone shape
Pillow	1 drop either side of pillow
Poultice	4 drops to 2 tablespoonsful of poultice base
Pulse point	1 drop to 1ml carrier oil
Room Air Spray	50 drops in 100ml pure water in garden spray or spray top bottle

Skin Oil / Lotion Cream /Ointment	1 drop for each 2ml (body), 4ml (facial)
Sitz Bath	3-4 dropsin a bowl large enough to sit in, filled with cool/warm water
Tissue / Hankie	1-2 drops direct on cloth
Vapouriser	6-8 drops in saucer of water (candle lit) 6-8 drops direct in electric

NORMAL SKIN: Lavender, Geranium, Rosemary, Rosewood, Evening Primrose, Sweet Orange, Cedarwood.
DRY SKIN: Lavender, Sandalwood, Geranium, Cedarwood, Rosewood, Ylang Ylang, Patchouli, Evening Primrose, Frankincense.
OILY SKIN: Cypress, Cedarwood, Lavender, Bergamot, Rosemary, Lemon, Sweet Orange, Juniper, Frankincense, Clary Sage, Lemongrass.
MATURE SKIN: Frankincense, Ylang Ylang, Sandalwood, Rosewood, Patchouli, Fennel, Lavender, Geranium, Cypress, Evening Primrose.
BLEMISHED SKIN: Rosemary, Lavender, Teatree, Lemon, Geranium.
SENSITIVE SKIN: Lavender, Sandalwood, Cedarwood, Evening Primrose.

Ailment	Oil	Adult Dosage (over 12 years)	Application
BACKACHE (Temporary Relief of Pain)	LAVENDER ROSEMARY JUNIPER	2 Drops each	Add to warm bath.
		1 Drop each	Warm compress to area.
		2 Drops each	Massage.Add to lOml. Base oil.
BITES/STINGS (Bee / Flea / Wasp / Mosquito)	TEA TREE LAVENDER	1 Drop of either	Neat. Topical application.
		2 Drops of each	Cold compress to area.
BRUISES	LAVENDER FENNEL CYPRESS	2 Drops each	Immediate ice-cold compress.
	ROSEMARY	2-3 Drops	Gentle massage when colour appears. in 5m1 Base oil.
BURNS (Minor)	LAVENDER	Neat as required	Immediately apply neat to affected area. Apply iced water or ice cold compress.
COLD & FLU (Temporary Relief of Symptoms)	LEMON PEPPERMINT EUCALYPTUS	4 Drops Combination	On tissue: use as required to clear head.
	LAVENDER TEA TREE EUCALYPTUS LEMON	6 Drops Combination of three	Vapouriser: During day to combat germs.
	PEPPERMINT ROSEMARY TEA TREE EUCALYPTUS	2 Drops Combination of two	Inhalation: During day as decongestant.
	LAVENDER GERANIUM MAJORAM	6-8 Drop Combination	Bath: In evening to aid sleep.
	LA\'ENDER EUCALYPTUS CEDARWOOD	4-6 Drops Combination in 5-lOml Base oil	Chest Back Rub: Before bed or during day.
COLD SORES (Relief of Symptoms)	GERANIUM TEA TREE	Neat: 1 Drop	On cotton bud. Apply to affected area as soon as tingling of skin starts.
CRAMPS (Relief of Pain)	MARJORAM CYPRESS GERANIUM	3-4 Drop Combination in 5ml Base oil	Massage: For leg cramps Warm Compress: To abdomen and Leg.
CUTS & GRAZES	LAVENDER LEMON TEA TREE EUCALYPTUS	6-10 Drops Combination or any single type. Add to I lt. boiled water	Bathe: To cleanse and sterilise. Leave wound uncovered if possible or add 1 drop Lavender neat to plaster.
NOTE: SEEK MEDICAL ATTENTION IF CUT IS DEEP OR BLOOD LOSS SIGNIFICANT			

EARACHE	LAVENDER	1 Drop	Neat: Apply to cotton wool and gently place in outer ear and dab behind ear. Warm Compress: Hot water bottle.
FEVER (Temporary Relief of Symptoms)	PEPPERMINT EUCALYPTUS BERGAMOT LAVENDER LEMONGRASS	1 Drop of Combination of 3	Tepid/Cool Compress: Apply to feet, arms and forehead. Add to bowl tepid water and sponge body. (NB: Lemongrass: Caution on skin).
WARNING: DRINK PLENTY OF FLUIDS & ALWAYS CONSULT A DOCTOR IF SYMPTOMS PERSIST.			
HANGOVER (Relief of Symptoms)	FENNEL JUNIPER ROSEMARY	2 Drops each in 10ml Carrier oil	Massage: circular motion to liver area.
		1 Drop each	Cold Compress: To head and back of neck.
HAYFEVER (Relief of Symptoms)	PEPPERMINT LEMON ROSEMARY LAVENDER CLOVE GERANIUM EUCALYPTUS	4 Drop Combination 3	Tissue: Inhale as required
		5 Drops/l0 ml Base oil	Massage: Neck, chest and back.
		6 Drops Combination3	Vapouriser: To clear atmosphere
NOTE: HAYFEVER AFFECTS PEOPLE IN DIFFERENT WAYS SO EXPERIMENT WITH THE ABOVE OILS TO SELECT THE BEST FOR YOU.			

HEADACHE (Temporary Relief of Symptoms)	PEPPERMINT ROSEMARY EUCALYPTUS LEMON	3 Drops Combination3	Inhalation: To help sinus headache
	BASIL GERANIUM LAVENDER CLARY SAGE MARJORAM	4-6 Drops Combination of 3 in Base oil	Massage: Scalp, neck and shoulders for tension headache.
	LAVENDER TEA TREE EUCALYPTUS PEPPERMINT LEMON	4-6 Drop Combination	Cold Compress: Apply to temples and neck.
		4 Drops	Tissue: Inhale when required.
		2 Drops	Pillow: To help sleep.
INSOMNIA (Relief of)	LAVENDER ORANGE MARJORAM CLARY SAGE FRANKINCENSE SANDALWOOD YLANG YLANG	10 Drop Combination of 3 in 20ml Carrier oil	Massage: Before bed.
		2 Drops of one.	Pillow: A drop each side.
		6-8 Drops Combination of 3	Bath: Before bed.
MENSTRUATION (Relief of Pain)	CLARY SAGE JUNIPER YLANG YLANG MARJORAM	4-6 Drop Combination of 3 in l0ml Base oil	Massage: Clockwise over solar plexus, lower abdomen and lower back. Warm Compress: Applied to abdomen and lower back. (Use hot water bottle)
NOTE: SEEK MEDICAL ADVICE IF PAIN PERSISTS,			
MOUTH ULCERS	ORANGE CLOVE BUD TEA TREE	1 Drop of either	Apply to cotton bud and apply to area.
NAUSEA	PEPPERMINT ORANGE LEMON LAVENDER	2 Drops of one.	Tissue: Inhale as needed.

NOSEBLEEDS	LAVENDER CYPRESS	1 Drop each in ice cold water.	Cold Compress: (Hankie) to bridge of nose.
PIMPLES	LAVENDER LEMON	3 Drop Combination 3 in 5ml Base oil.	Dab on affected area with Cotton bud.
	TEA TREE PEPPERMINT	1 Drop neat	Dab on affected area with cotton bud

SUNBURN (Relief of Pain)	LAVENDER	2 Drops	Add to tub of natural yogurt, apply and cover with Cotton t-shirt.
	LAVENDER TEA TREE SANDALWOOD PEPPERMINT	4-6 Drop Combination in 10ml Jojoba	Bath: Tepid water to soothe and cool. Skin Oil: Smoothe over gently to nourish.
TOOTHACHE (Temporary Relief of Pain)	CLOVE PEPPERMINT TEA TREE	1 Drop	Apply to Cotton bud, dab on affected tooth or dilute in Base oil for children.(Avoid lips).
CAUTION: SEE DENTIST IF PAIN PERSISTS.			
WARTS	LEMON CLOVE LAVENDER	1 Drop of any	Apply to cotton bud. Dab direct on wart.

LEGEND:	
C = Compress	D = Direct Application
B = Bathe	**M = Massage**
T = Tissue	
Quick Reference Chart of Dosages	
Nature's Medicine Cabinet	

Bites	Lavender/Tea Tree	D
Blisters	Lavender/Tea Tree	D
Bruises	Geranium/Lavender	C
Bumps	Lavender	C
Chills	Geranium	C B
Colds	Eucalyptus/Peppermint	**M** T
Cuts	Lavender/Eucalyptus/Tea Tree	B
Cramps	Geranium	C **M**
Fever	Eucalyptus/Lavender	C B
Hayfever	Eucalyptus/Peppermint/Lavender/Geranium	**M** T
Headache	Peppermint/Lavender	C **M** T
Heat Exhaustion	Lavender/Eucalyptus	C B
Insect Repellent	Lavender/Peppermint/Eucalyptus/Tea Tree/Geranium	**M**

Muscle Aches	Lavender/Eucalyptus	C B **M**
Rashes	Geranium/Eucalyptus/Lavender	C B
Sleeplessness	Lavender/Geranium	C B **M**
Sunburn	Lavender/Peppermint/Eucalyptus	B **M**
Travel Sickness	Peppermint	C T
Toothache	Peppermint/Tea Tree	D
Vomiting	Peppermint/Lavender	C T
Upset Tummy	Lavender/Peppermint	C **M** T

Effect	Lemon	Sweet Marjoram	Orange	Peppermint	Rose	Rosemary	Sandalwood	Tea-Tree	Ylang Ylang
anti-bacterial	X	X					X	X	
anti-inflammation	X			X		X		X	
anti-rheumatic		X				X			
anti-spasmodic		X		X		X	X		
anti-viral	X			X				X	
asthma		X					X		
bronchitis		X		X		X	X	X	
calming		X	X		X		X		X
colds	X	X		X		X			
depression		X			X	X	X		X
disinfect air	X	X		X		X			
energize				X		X			
fatigue				X		X			
fevers	X					X		X	

Effect	Lemon	Sweet Marjoram	Orange	Peppermint	Rose	Rosemary	Sandalwood	Tea-Tree	Ylang Ylang
headache/migraine		X		X		X			
hypertension	X	X							X
insomnia		X	X		X		X		X
meditation							X		
menstrual cramps		X		X		X			
menopause					X				
mental acuity				X		X			
muscle stress		X				X			
nervousness	X	X	X				X		X
pms		X							

pain relief		X		X		X			
stress		X	X		X		X		X
wounds/burns								X	

- When pregnant avoid Atlas Cedar, Basil, Clary Sage, Juniper, Marjoram, Peppermint & Rosemary.
- Clary Sage should be avoided if you have endometriosis, breast, ovarian or uterine cysts, estrogen dependent conditions (cancers).
- Avoid Rosemary if you have high blood pressure or
- epilepsy. Peppermint and Lemon may irritate sensitive skin.
- Bergamot, Lemon and Orange may cause skin sensitivity to the sun.

Traditional Therapeutic Effects of Ancient Healing Art Blends These tables cross reference the traditional therapeutic effects of the nine Ancient Healing Art Essential Oil Blends This reference table was created to make choosing a blend (that is just right for you) easier.

headache/migraine							X		X
insomnia					X		X	X	
meditation					X				
menstrual cramps			X						
menopause	X								
muscle stress				X					
pms	X							X	
pain relief	X	X	X	X					
stress	X			X	X	X	X	X	

REFLEXOLOGY AND AROMATHERAPY BIBLE By Toni Austin

- When pregnant avoid Energizer, Northwest Comfort, Muscle Relief, Peace, Serenity and Vitality
- Northwest Comfort and Muscle Tension Relief should be avoided if you have endometriosis, breast, ovarian or uterine cysts or estrogen dependent conditions (cancers)

About the Author

Physical fitness has rarely witnessed such a perfect expression of grace, poise, style and strength as Ms Toni Austin, a living example of what can be achieved through the right combination of exercise and super-smart nutrition. Auburn-haired Toni hails from Texas and she just loves the great outdoors, the open spaces, the endless sky and the fresh air. As a child, she excelled at sports and was encouraged to follow a career as a fitness pro. She earned her first degree in physical education and, whilst still a student, fell in love with the Pilates exercise system. The Pilates method equipped her with a new range of techniques for helping people to maximise their fitness potential and her experience with Pilates led her to Yoga and an intensive course of study in India. Her training and dedication fully equipped her to become an exceptionally gifted Yoga teacher.

Toni's main ambition has always been to share her knowledge and experience with everyone she meets, helping people to get into better shape and discover the joys of natural fitness. But she also recognised that food also plays a major role in determining so many of our health issues. Always highly motivated to develop her professional knowledge, this was when she began studying nutritional science. Toni became a celebrated nutritional coach and the result has been an astonishing list of successes with individuals of all ages and backgrounds.

Toni understands the way our bodies really work. She knows first-hand that if you get the nutrition right and add the right kind of exercise, it really is possible to burn off the excess pounds, to master all weight issues and tame them forever. And that's a source of great satisfaction to her and to her clients. Combining her extensive experience as a fitness coach with her life-long passion for using smart nutrition and natural cures to enhance the quality of peoples' lives, Toni is the living, breathing example of vibrant health and youthful vigour.

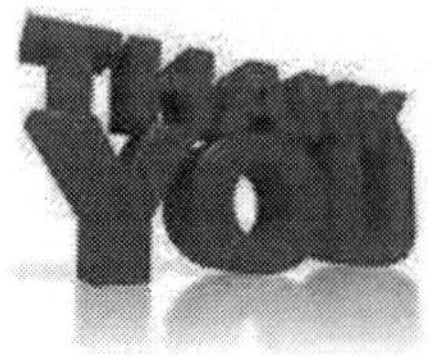

I am so delighted that you have chosen this book and it's been a pleasure writing it for you. My mission is to help as many readers as possible to benefit from the content you have just been reading. So many of us are able to take new information and apply it to our lives with really positive and long lasting consequences and it is my wish that you have been able to take value from the information I have presented Thank you for staying with me during this book and for reading it through to the end. I really hope that you have enjoyed the contents and that's why I appreciate your feedback so much. If you could take a couple of minutes to review the book, your views will help me to create more material that you find beneficial.

I am always delighted to hear from my readers and you can email me personally via the Publisher at the email address beranparry@gmail.com if you have any questions about this book or future books. Let us know how we can help you by sending a message to the same email address.

Thanks again for your support and encouragement. I really look forward to reading your review.

Stay Healthy!

Click Here to go to the review Page

FOR MORE BY
MERCEDES DEL REY

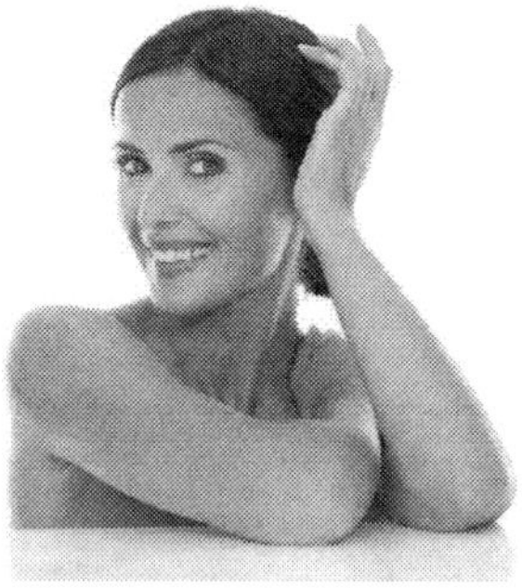

Please search thispage
https://www.amazon.com/s/ref=dp_byline_sr_ebooks_1?ie=UTF8&field-author=Mercedes+Del+Rey&search-alias=digital-text&text=Mercedes+Del+Rey&sort=relevancerank

Your Ultimate Herbal Miracle Manual
Your Permanent Handbook for Herbal Treatments
With this easy to use Herbal Miracle Manual, you will be able to:
*** Learn more about Herbs and Medicine
*** Find out how to use herbs to help some of your conditions
*** Improve your understanding of how herbs help us
*** Learn about which herbs help certain conditions
*** Broaden your understanding of the healing properties of herbs

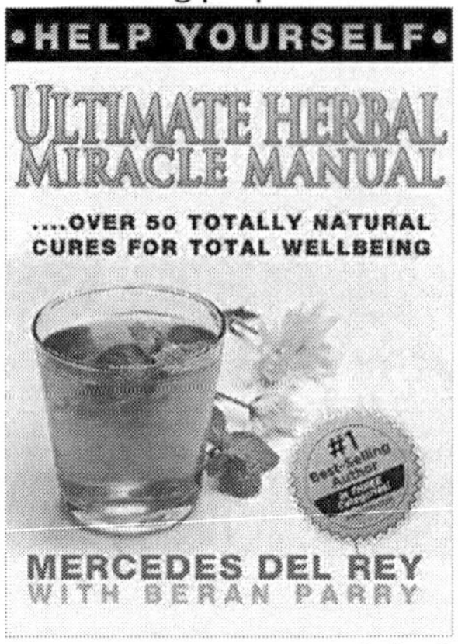

Please search the web site www.amazon.com/s/ref=nb_sb_noss?url=search-alias%3Ddigital-text&field-keywords=B0185HGFVC

The Ultimate Herbal Detox Tea Book
(Over 75 Herbal Tea Cures for Toxic Symptoms)
Your Permanent Detox Tea Handbook

Detoxing your body was never so simple or so tasty! If you feel that your health could use a helping hand, if your wellbeing could use a boost, download your copy of the Ultimate Herbal Tea Guide right now and sip your way gently to better health and a cleaner, happier body.

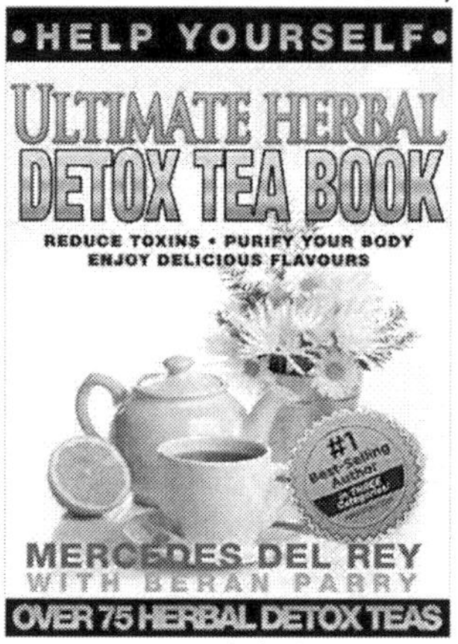

Please search this web site www.amazon.com/s/ref=nb_sb_noss?url=search-alias%3Ddigital-text&field-keywords=B019OSH1JG

From the Same Publisher
By Beran Parry
The Ultimate PALEO KETOGENIC Anti-Inflammatory Diet
Reduce Pain-Gain Energy
50 Delicious, Easy, Anti Inflammatory Paleo

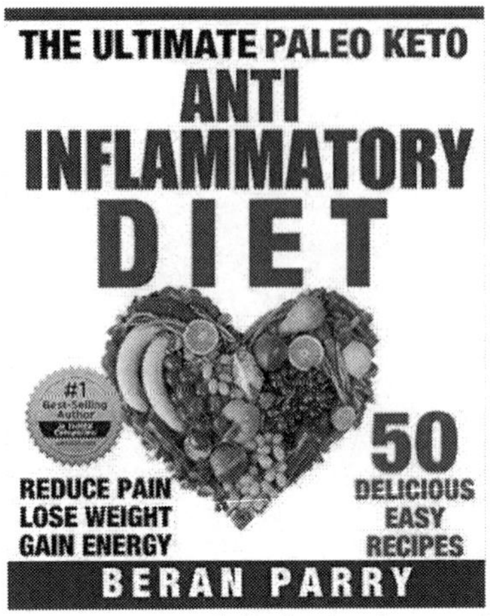

Please search this page www.amazon.com/s/ref=nb_sb_noss?url=search-alias%3Ddigital-text&field-keywords=B01DHQKTKY

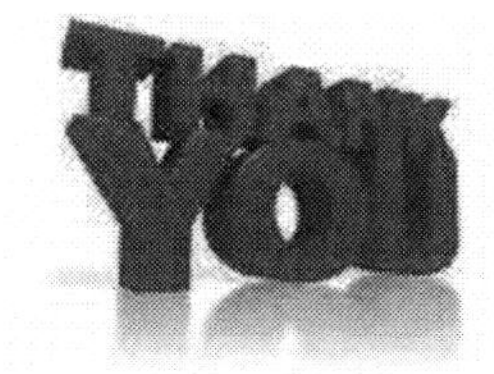

I am so delighted that you have chosen this book and it's been a pleasure writing it for you. My mission is to help as many readers as possible to benefit from the content you have just been reading. So many of us are able to take new information and apply it to our lives with really positive and long lasting consequences and it is my wish that you have been able to take value from the information I have presented

Thank you for staying with me during this book and for reading it through to the end. I really hope that you have enjoyed the contents and that's why I appreciate your feedback so much. If you could take a couple of minutes to review the book, your views will help me to create more material that you find beneficial.
I am always delighted to hear from my readers and you can email me via the publisher at beranparry@gmail.com if you have any questions about this book or future books. Let us know how we can help you by sending a message to the same email address.
Thanks again for your support and encouragement. I really look forward to reading your review.
Stay Healthy!
Click Here to go to the review Page

60282875R00060

Made in the USA
Middletown, DE
28 December 2017